THE MEMORY CURE

The Safe, Scientifically Proven Breakthrough That Can Slow, Halt, or Even Reverse Age-Related Memory Loss

Millions of Americans, in their mid-forties or beyond, have experienced some degree of memory loss. Now, Dr. Thomas H. Crook III, one of America's leading experts on memory impairment, and bestselling author and medical researcher Brenda Adderly present a cutting-edge solution to age-related forgetfulness. *THE MEMORY CURE* is an accessible, six-step program that incorporates the powers of phosphatidylserine, or PS, a dietary supplement derived from the soybean, which has been scientifically tested and proven safe and effective—and which offers new hope and vibrant mental acuity to all who have felt their memory slipping away. Discover:

- why we become forgetful as we age
- how PS works—and how to reap its greatest benefits in a total lifestyle plan for curbing memory loss
- surprising dietary sources of PS
- Memory Maximizer exercises that are effective and fun
- other natural memory boosters, including fish, ginkgo biloba, ginseng, antioxidants, trace minerals such as boron and zinc, and vitamins
- new information on the impact of certain drugs and diseases on memory
- how to prevent memory failure before it starts . . . and much more!

ALSO BY THOMAS CROOK
How to Remember Names

ALSO BY BRENDA ADDERLY (coauthor)
The Arthritis Cure
The Fat Blocker Diet
The Complete Guide to Pills
Maximizing the Arthritis Cure
The Pain Relief Breakthrough
The Arthritis Cure Cookbook
Brighter Baby
The Doctors' Guide to Over-the-Counter Drugs
The Prostate Cure

THE
MEMORY
CURE

THOMAS H. CROOK III, Ph.D.,
& BRENDA ADDERLY, M.H.A.

POCKET BOOKS
New York   London   Toronto   Sydney   Tokyo   Singapore

POCKET BOOKS, a division of Simon & Schuster Inc.
1230 Avenue of the Americas, New York, NY 10020

ISBN: 0-671-02643-7

First Pocket Books paperback printing June 1999

10 9 8 7 6 5 4 3 2 1

Cover design by Mike Stromberg

Text design by Stanley S. Drate/Folio Graphics Co. Inc.

Printed in the U.S.A.

To my late grandfather, Raymond Hunter, with deep gratitude for so many wonderful childhood memories.

—THOMAS CROOK

To my husband, Peter Engel, and our two boys who are on the way—here's to creating great memories for the coming adventure!

—BRENDA ADDERLY

ACKNOWLEDGMENTS

We first owe a debt of gratitude to Howard Cohl, Peter Engel, Jeffry Still, Sandra Thompson, and everyone at Affinity for their support, hard work, understanding, and encouragement during this very "memorable" project.

Then, we would like to thank Parris Kidd, Ph.D., most sincerely for his contributions to our understanding of phosphatidylserine (PS). Much of the technical material in this book is based on the work of Dr. Kidd, although the conclusions drawn in the text are ours.

We would also like to thank Peter Rohde and Jens Heiser, the CEOs of Lucas Meyer, USA, and the Lucas Meyer parent company in Germany, respectively, for making copious information about the supplement available to us. We have not always conformed precisely with their views, but we have always found them valuable.

Finally, we would like to thank our incredible editor, Nancy Miller, for her guidance, fortitude, and extraordinary faith that we would get the manuscript completed on time. That we managed to do so is largely due to the fact that we could not let her down!

CONTENTS

AN IMPORTANT NOTE
TO OUR READERS

The material in this book is for informational purposes only. It is not intended to serve as a prescription for you, or to replace the advice of your medical doctor. Please discuss all aspects of the Memory Cure with your physician *before* beginning any program. If you have any medical conditions, or are taking prescription or non-prescription medications, see your physician before altering or discontinuing the use of them.

Why Do We Use the Word "Cure"?

Our use of the word *cure* is substantiated by several references. We use the word cure to mean the partial or complete relief of the symptoms of a memory that is declining because of age. Obviously, nothing in the title or content of this book is intended to suggest that the use of the recommended supplements or program will fully restore such a failing memory. Moreover, we make it quite clear that our "cure" only applies to age-associated memory impairment (AAMI), which is technically not a disease at all. We are not in any way suggesting that our recommendations will significantly help cure or even restore a memory lost or diminished as a result of: Alzheimer's disease, any other disease, prescription drugs, or accidental brain damage. The evidence, carefully collected in this book, fully substantiates that, for AAMI, the supplements recommended are frequently effective for long periods of time. However, we offer no guarantee that *every* individual will benefit from this program.

THE
MEMORY
CURE

1

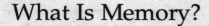

What Is Memory?

The dimension of the problem

What causes memory to decline?

Memory loss classified

The structures of the brain

What is memory?

*What type of age-associated memory
impairment (AAMI) needs to be cured?*

Retrieval versus recall

Summary

Janice was upset and embarrassed. She frequently forgot appointments, and sometimes, in the middle of a sentence, she forgot what she was going to say. Only 58

years old, Janice worried that she was in the first throes of Alzheimer's disease.

Norman, in his early sixties, was concerned because more and more he found himself saying, "I know it; I know it . . . Give me a minute and it will come to me."

Typically, memory loss starts gradually. We slowly become aware that we aren't remembering as well as we used to. As time passes, however, we begin to forget important things so frequently that we can no longer ignore it. Yet none of our other faculties are impaired. We still have no problems walking, holding intelligent conversations, or enjoying concerts. So why are we having this increasingly frustrating and deeply worrying experience?

When it works well, remembering seems almost instinctual, something we take for granted. We tend to think of it as always with us, ever reliable, until that disconcerting moment when it betrays us: We're at an exciting party. Having had a couple of drinks, we turn to a new acquaintance to introduce our best friend, whom we've known since college, and—can't remember her last name. It's never happened before; it may not even have happened to you . . . yet.

However, the fact that you purchased *The Memory Cure* says that you have some concern about the workings of your memory or that of someone you love. Rest assured, you are not alone. A brief review of the term "memory" on the Internet shows hundreds of sites concerned with various topics related to memory. Most have "brain-boosting" courses, tapes, or software they want to sell you. Others advocate herbs or supplements that purport to improve your memory. But only a few have any up-to-date information on memory research, and none that we have found bring you the full body of accurate information you need to deal with this problem.

A memory that is starting to fail is not something most of us are able to shrug off as "just one of those things" that happens as we get older. On the contrary, memory is vital to our lives. Its decline is both annoying for the things we forget, and, for most people, very disturbing for the serious problems it may portend. Without a doubt, memory loss is one of *the* most terrifying aspects of aging.

If you feel you are starting to lose your ability to learn and remember, you're not alone. Millions of aging Americans have similar experiences and similar concerns. Until recently, virtually no one believed that there was a serious, practical, effective treatment for a failing memory. Even today, few people know that such a treatment does, in fact, exist, although many European doctors have been using it for more than a decade.

Many physicians will tell you there's nothing you can do about aging and accompanying memory loss. But that is incorrect. In fact, it can be delayed or even restored by using a *safe, scientifically proven, clinically tested natural food supplement* that is available without a prescription in most health food stores in the United States.

The Dimension of the Problem

How big a problem is age-associated memory impairment (AAMI) really? Whom does it affect? How much does memory decline? And is it a precursor to Alzheimer's so that we can all expect to descend into that gray world of dementia if we are "lucky" enough to survive cancer, heart attacks, and assorted accidents and thus manage to live to an otherwise healthy old age?

These are vitally important questions to which almost everyone reaching or passing middle age wants answers. For those answers will, after all, have a determinant influence on the rest of our lives.

Until recently, memory loss was something we recognized intuitively but had not measured. However, in the last few years, research conducted by Dr. Thomas Crook (the coauthor of this book) and others has made accurate answers available. No longer do we have to rely on our feeling that our memories are declining; now we know the quality and dimension of that decline. And, in knowing those facts, we are at last able to do something about them.

Baldly stated, in the absence of any curative solution, the steady decline in memory in otherwise reasonably healthy people as they age is very substantial. While that sounds depressing, there are three pieces of very good news:

◆ Below advanced old age, say age 85 or more, the incidence of memory declining so far as to be classified as Alzheimer's disease (AD) is low. Probably less than 10 percent of the 75- to 85-year-old population suffers from AD; less than 5 percent of 65- to 75-year-olds show symptoms of the disease; and only a tiny percentage of people under 65 can be diagnosed as having AD. And even above 85 years, when, after all, for most people nearly all physical and mental systems weaken and break down, at least two-thirds of us do not have and will *never* get AD.

◆ Even more fortunately, the nutritional supplement on which this book is focused will substantially reduce ordinary memory loss. It will do this both by delaying the loss so that it happens at a later age, and by reducing the absolute amount of memory capacity that is ever lost. Indeed, for many people, this supplement will significantly reverse memory losses that have already occurred. We cover this remarkable supplement and the results it achieves in full detail in Chapter 3.

◆ Finally, the other five steps of the memory cure described in this book will further reverse the absolute loss of memory at any age, and/or help readers to improve their memory so much that, for all practical purposes, their total *effective* memory need not decline at all. Indeed, in many cases, it is likely to be significantly enhanced.

Thus, the overall message of this book is that you can largely or entirely overcome the problem of AAMI with a nutritional supplement coupled with an easy-to-implement plan we call the Memory Maximizer.

Before we deal with the methods of how to overcome AAMI, however, we should first define the dimension of the problem we are seeking to solve. For, while it was generally recognized until the early 1990s that there is a decline in memory performance associated with normal aging, there was considerable disagreement about how severe this decline was. However, today we have a variety of detailed long-term studies to tell us more precisely the dimension of the problem we face.

◆ In 1991, Youngjohn, Larrabee, and Crook tested 1,535 healthy, normal subjects on their ability to learn and remember written information. The chart shows that, in this respect, there is a decline from age 25 to age 40–49 of 21 percent, and that this decline continues, so that by age 70–79, the decline has reached 43 percent (Fig. 1.1).[1]

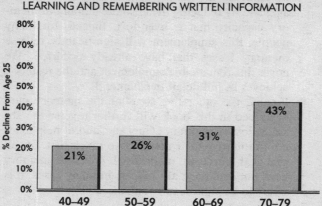

Fig. 1.1: DECLINE IN MEMORY WITH ADVANCING AGE
LEARNING AND REMEMBERING WRITTEN INFORMATION

◆ In 1993 a team of nine researchers under the guidance of Dr. Crook published the results of a definitive study on how age affects memory, testing 908 subjects for 90 minutes each with a sophisticated computerized test battery and organizing the mountain of data they obtained so that it could be thoroughly analyzed. The subjects were chosen from a random sampling of the population of the Republic of San Marino on the Italian peninsula.[2]

The results showed a comparable major decline. For example, respondents were tested on their ability to remember names immediately and then one hour after introduction. In immediate recall, as compared to age 25, there was a 29 percent decline by age 40–49 and a remarkable 65 percent decline by age 70–79. An hour later, the situation had become even worse, with declines from age 25 to age 40–49 of 35 percent and 74 percent to age 70–79 (Fig. 1.2).

In all, Dr. Crook et al. have conducted more than twenty major studies of various types of memory decline and they all show a similar pattern. Moreover, these findings are consistent with the observations of virtually every other researcher in the field and with the more subjective experience of almost every practitioner who deals regularly with the elderly.

The sad fact is that, left unattended, our memories decline substantially with age. And that decline can cause a serious reduction in our effectiveness as we get older, hence in the quality of our lives. Happily, however, as we shall show in this book, today that problem can be largely or entirely eliminated.

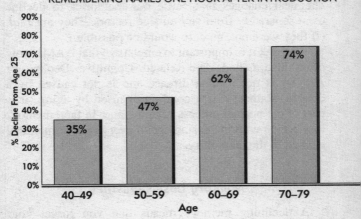

Fig. 1.2: DECLINE IN MEMORY WITH ADVANCING AGE
REMEMBERING NAMES ONE HOUR AFTER INTRODUCTION

What Causes Memory to Decline?

In order to solve the problem of memory decline, we first need to understand its causes. Until recently we knew surprisingly little about them. However, today our knowledge and understanding of how memory works—and why it declines—has been greatly advanced. Although we don't yet have all the answers, we do know that, contrary to what you may have heard, aging and memory loss do not depend solely on how long our parents lived nor on any preset, mystical time line. Rather, a variety of factors impinging on our busy lives, such as stress, disorganization, and lack of concentration or attention, interfere with our ability to remember important facts. Indeed, part of the reason that our memories worsen with age is that these outside factors become stronger and more disruptive. We have more to do, more pressures upon us, more information to sift, store, and recall. But that is clearly only part of the problem. The chemical changes that cause our memories to decline exist separately from any outside factors. They are *real*. (If they were not, no cure would be possible.)

We think it is important to emphasize that AAMI (now often also called Age-Related Cognitive Decline or ARCD) is not itself a disease and is not caused by a disease. Rather, it is a condition caused by aging. It is part of the normal process of aging and, in fact, memory loss occurs with increasing age in every type of mammal studied in the laboratory.

Memory Loss Classified

A declining memory means that you forget your friend's e-mail address, or the name of that movie you saw last week and want to recommend to someone. While these are not trivial, they are merely annoying lapses you can learn to live with. For example, you can carry your ATM number with you, appropriately concealed, of course. In fact, most of us take these small pieces of forgetfulness for granted. If that were all there was to memory decline, it wouldn't be such a worry. Far worse, however, are the memory lapses that reduce our ability to live our lives as we wish.

"I have to read every book twice to recall it," a 60-year-old woman, who recently returned to college to study history, complained. "When I was younger, one good skim through was enough."

Similarly, as we age we do less well on "source memory," remembering where we got certain information. Thus, we have more trouble than younger persons in distinguishing whether some facts are true or illusory. Cognitive psychologist Daniel Schacter and his colleagues made up some juicy tidbits of gossip. They told old and young participants that some were secrets that should not be disclosed and that others were common knowledge. Older adults had more difficulty remembering which were the secrets and which were not.[3]

Brenda Adderly (the other coauthor of this book) remembers the experience of a close friend with a virtually infallible memory, whom we will call Kenneth. As a college student, and later as a businessman, Kenneth never took notes. He simply remembered everything he heard. As he explains it, "I couldn't understand how anyone could forget things."

Then shortly after his fifty-fifth birthday, he had an experience that was terrifying for him. "As usual," Kenneth says, "I had attended several meetings the prior day, and I recalled that one in particular required me to follow up on it. *But I couldn't remember what I was supposed to do.* I was horrified. I thought I was losing my mind," he recalls.

Although reassured by others, including his own doctor, Kenneth had slammed against a wall he feared was mental decline. "I was afraid it was all downhill from there," he says, "and I was terrified to think where it would end."

Kenneth was about to learn that to compensate for their reduced memory, older people can simply work a little harder. They can take more notes, write more detailed lists, and confirm everything in writing. Of course, while these techniques are useful to compensate, they cannot cure AAMI.

Kenneth's memory today, 15 years later, is still strong. But it is noticeably weaker than it was. If Kenneth had been experiencing this problem now instead of a decade ago, this would not be the case. His memory would have declined far less, if at all. And today, we can stop his memory declining further—and perhaps even help him to reverse some of the extant decline.

Indeed, the astounding truth is that a failing memory is no longer an inevitable fact of aging. It *can* be halted, reversed, and even effectively cured, and *The Memory Cure* will show you how. The findings reported in this book reveal that, for healthy people whose memory decline is due to aging, and not caused by a stroke or some other illness, taking the nutritional supplement recommended in Chapter 3 and following the memory maximizing plan recommended in Chapter 4 will help maintain or even regain a high measure of cognitive brain function, including the ability to:

◆ remember names of persons to whom you are introduced

◆ recognize faces
◆ remember easily forgotten details such as names and telephone numbers
◆ recall accurately the content of conversations and professional discussions
◆ learn and remember new information
◆ maintain a high level of concentration
◆ improve verbal ability

Memory is not a simple "thing." It is complex, multi-faceted, and fascinating, as is the brain itself.

The Structures of the Brain

There are many subdivisions of the brain, and it may perhaps be helpful to review some of them briefly to fully understand how the brain works. This will, of course, have a bearing on how memory and age-related forgetting occur. However, some of you may already be familiar with the structure of the brain, and others may lack a bent for anatomy and may be intimidated. In either case, please feel free to jump ahead to the section, "What Is Memory?"

Scientists believe that the oldest parts of our brain, the *brainstem* and *midbrain,* developed more than 500 million years ago. They are the first parts of our brain to be formed in the womb. Because they resemble the entire brain of a reptile, they are sometimes called the "reptilian brain." Sitting atop our spinal column, they determine our level of alertness, and handle such automatic and basic bodily functions as breathing and heart rate.

Scientists believe that before "bundles" of new information are stored as memory, they temporarily reside in a structure called the *hippocampus,* a horseshoe-shaped structure buried deep in the brain above the ear.[4]

For the last quarter of a century, the hippocampus has been intensively investigated. So important is this area that it even has a journal (appropriately titled *Hippocampus*) dedicated to research about it. Studies conducted during the last decade with laboratory monkeys have further identified the structures within the hippocampal region, including adjacent areas linked to it, that are important for memory. We do know that the hippocampus is involved in the recognition of newness[5] and helps "decide" whether important facts and events will be stored in the brain permanently. New memories are initially dependent on the hippocampal system and its adjacent areas,[6] but they gradually become established in other areas of the brain.[7] After the age of forty, the hippocampus loses a small percentage of its cells each year, accounting for some of the memory problems that occur with aging.

An extreme case of what happens as a result of such a cellular decline is Frank, who sustained severe injuries in a car accident. He can understand directions on how to accomplish a new task he has never done before and, with repeated instruction, he can accomplish that task. However, if he is asked to repeat the same task the next day, he will be quite unable to do so. He has learned nothing. That is because, with a damaged hippocampus, Frank can still comprehend incoming information, and understand what is being said, but he cannot hold on to the information for any length of time.

The hippocampus plays an especially important role in processing and remembering spatial and contextual information[8] such as the route to your best friend's house or the golf course. Thank your hippocampus the next time you don't get lost. Blame it, as you age, if you find yourself taking a wrong turn when you knew the right one perfectly well.

It is via the hippocampus that our brains have a communication link with the immune system and with our emotional memory. It seems that the cells of the hippocampus and the cortex (see page 14) are some of the continually busiest cells in the body.

THE LITTLE BRAIN AND ITS COMPANION, THE CEREBRUM

Attached to the rear of your brainstem is the *cerebellum* ("little brain"), located at the back of your head just above the neck. It adjusts posture, coordinates muscular movement, and stores the memories of simple learned movements. We use this part of our brain so much that it has more than tripled in size during the last million years of human development, but it still isn't the largest part of the brain. That's the *cerebrum.*

Gradually developing over the past 200 million years, the cerebrum is divided into two halves or hemispheres, each of which controls the opposite side of the body. The hemispheres are connected by the *corpus callosum,* a band of some 300 million nerve fibers, which tends to be larger in females. The cerebrum permits us to develop our two most prominent and distinct ways of thinking: verbally/logically (left side) and visually/spatially (right side).

A one-eighth-inch-thick, intricately folded layer of nerve cells covers the cerebrum. Called the *cortex* (Latin for "bark"), it is the most recently evolved portion of the brain. The cortex, which could cover about two and a half feet if stretched out, is very convoluted and shaped by ridges and grooves.

Among its other functions, the cortex allows us to re-

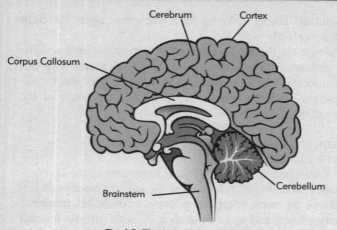

***Fig. 1.3:* The Major Parts of the Brain**
Over 200 million years of evolution have created our most complex organ.

member, to analyze and compare incoming information with stored information, to organize experiences, to learn to speak a language, and to make decisions. Without it, we would exist in a vegetative state, although still alive because the other parts of the brain take care of that.

With age, it appears that there may be a very gradual shrinking of the cortex. (Ironically, it becomes less wrinkled just as our faces are doing the opposite!) AAMI results, in part, from this shrinking. Perhaps we cannot entirely avoid this cortical change but, as we shall show, we may be able to delay it with the supplement this book recommends, and to compensate for the shrinking in other ways as well.

The cortex of each hemisphere is divided into four areas called *lobes.* Specific areas of the cortex and its lobes are devoted to the temporary processing of different sensory functions, and the type of information you're receiving determines which part of your brain is active. We know this from "pictures" or scans that have been taken of brains actively performing specific tasks.

The largest of the four lobes, the *frontal lobes,* has been associated with the performance of higher-level cognitive functions such as organization. They have the "executive" control of a number of complex mental processes. The frontal lobes allow us to make plans, control and focus our attention, make decisions, solve problems, and engage in purposeful behavior. They are particularly important for storing past events. Early research with monkeys, called upon to remember under which of two covers a piece of food has been hidden, indicated that it was the prefrontal cortex of the brain that was active during the problem-solving.

Injury or damage to the frontal lobe can leave a person easily distracted and unable to focus attention. In comparing older persons with younger patients who had le-

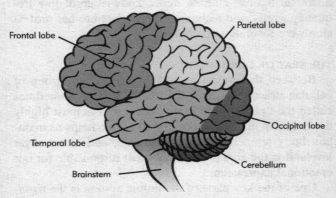

Fig. 1.4: The Four Lobes of the Brain
Each lobe processes different sensory functions like vision, memory, and abstract reasoning.

sions in their frontal lobes, Canadian researchers were able to show that at least some of the cognitive decline in their group of older persons matched that of younger, damaged patients and was likely due, therefore, to frontal system dysfunction.[9]

The *parietal lobes* extend up from the ear to the top of the head. They receive the information we take in from touch, and are partly involved in memory expression for up to at least two months.[10] The *occipital lobes,* located at the very back of the head and sometimes called the visual cortex, are responsible for vision. The *temporal lobes,* which fit under the temporal bone above the ears, are involved with hearing, perception, and language-generated memory (also called semantic and general memory).[11] When a 56-year-old Japanese woman developed lesions in the left temporal lobe of her brain following surgery, her language and autobiographic memory were preserved. Yet her semantic memory for public events, historical figures, cultural items, knowledge of low frequency words, and technical terms related to her profession were severely impaired.[12]

THE SEAT OF OUR EMOTIONS

Between the brainstem and the cortex is a group of cellular structures called the *limbic system.* Sometimes called the "mammalian brain" because it is most highly developed in mammals, our limbic system helps us maintain body temperature, heartbeat rate, and blood sugar levels. It is the area of the brain most responsible for our emotional expression.

One of the key parts of the limbic system is the *hypothalamus.* It directs those emotional reactions that have to do with survival (the "fight or flight" syndrome). By controlling hormonal secretions of the pituitary and by regulating the activity of the autonomic nervous system, the hypothalamus plays a critical role in enabling us to cope with stressful events. However, as we age, our reaction to stress tends to change. Some of us become more frightened and "stressed out," but many older people are calmer, less likely to want to fight or flee. While no one knows how such increased placidity may affect our memory, one possibility is that our relative lack of hypothalamic arousal may cause our memories to be less fully activated, thus giving the appearance that they are less powerful as we age.

The *amygdala* (a-MIG-duh-la), another part of our limbic system, is an almond-shaped structure situated in the temporal lobe just in front of the hippocampus. Along with the hippocampus, the amygdala helps transfer information from short-term to long-term memory. However, its main function seems to be that of linking memories that were formed through several senses. Thus, when you register the sight, sound, and smell of the ocean, along with the taste of salt on your lips, the amygdala is busy at work processing that input. The amygdala also plays a vital role in our emotional memories, including the development of memories about unpleasant experiences, which can develop into continuing fears or phobias.

What Is Memory?

Memory is complicated; the theories about it range far and wide; the literature covering it is copious enough to fill a good-sized library; and, with all that, no one yet has all the answers. Your potential to remember began, of course, when you were born, but your memory ability took a great spurt when you were about eight months old. It was then that you had enough experience and brain growth to begin to develop what child psychologists call "active memory"; that is, the ability to retrieve the past, to hold it in the present, and to simultaneously compare and relate new or incoming information with that past knowledge. It's a skill you continued to develop and to bring into your adult life. It allows you to find connections between "pieces" of experience. That ability to continue to make memories and new connections during your lifetime has led cognitive researchers to believe that the brain actually has more plasticity—that certain neurons can change structurally or functionally—than they previously thought.

Do you remember learning to remember? Of course not. But you did. It's one of those abilities we take for granted and presume we've always had. In truth, you spent the latter part of your first year of life developing and practicing your active memory skills. By the time you were seven or eight years old, your ability to retain information for a short time was about as good as that of your parents, but it was not until you were 12 or 13 that your memory capabilities approached theirs.

Once you reached adulthood, and certainly by middle age, your memory started to decline. Gradually, this worrying phenomenon has been studied and understood. As a result, in addition to knowing that we lose memory capacity over time, we also know what parts of it we lose, and recently we have found ways largely to compensate for those losses. Therefore, before we show you how to cure a memory that is declining due to age, we must first define the key components of that memory and describe how they work. So to the task . . .

Memory can, most usefully, be defined from three separate perspectives: over time; by content; and by the process of its formation. Let us cover each of these in turn.

OVER TIME

There are four reasonably separate types of memory over time:

◆ **Immediate Memory.** This is the sort of memory that lets you look up an unknown telephone number, dial it, and then forget it. Many of us cannot remember even the whole number. We look up the first part, dial it, and forget it; then look up the second half, dial it, and forget it in turn. But even if you can remember the entire number long enough to punch it out on your telephone, if you are like most people you will have to repeat the whole process if you need to repeat the call even a minute or two later.

Naturally, people vary with what they remember short term. A friend of ours cannot dial a telephone number without remembering it for hours; but he will forget a new word he reads (unless he is concentrating, of course) in an instant.

We humans can only be conscious and aware of a limited number of items at any single moment. For most of us, our short-term memory can only contain seven "chunks" or bunches of information, plus or minus two, an amount first determined by psychologist George A. Miller.[13] This means that we can think about or hold on to about seven different things or ideas at the same time. For instance, the letters S-E-E-C-I-A-C-B-S can either be thought of as nine different chunks (hard for most people to memorize), or as the three chunks SEE, CIA, and CBS (much easier to memorize, wouldn't you agree?).

◆ **Short-term Memory.** "Concentrating." That is the key. If we hear or read a telephone number or a word that is important to us, we imprint it into our minds and remember it beyond the "immediate" term and into the short run. Alternatively, if we are exposed to the same piece of information—even a trivial one—often enough, it too becomes imprinted. In either case, having entered our short-term memory bank, the information stays with us for minutes or hours. Nevertheless, the information is essentially temporary: We are not particularly interested in remembering it next week, and we are not likely to.

While the novice chess player may be able to think only one or two moves ahead in the game, grand masters can think at least seven to nine moves ahead at any one time. In one recall experiment, a chess master was able to reproduce nine boards from memory with more than 70 percent average accuracy, replacing as many as 160 pieces correctly.[14] Clearly, that would have been beyond the capacity of most casual players. But that is not necessarily because they have poorer memories. Rather, it is because, for such players, the location of chess pieces is not very important and therefore penetrates only as far as their short-term memory, whereas for a grand master this information is viewed as important enough to be long term.

◆ **Long-term Memory.** Some of the information we assimilate short term is sufficiently important or repeated often enough to become part of our "permanent" memory bank. Thus, it becomes part of "everything we know." This long-term memory, then, encompasses the main portions of our education, our recognition of friends and locations, our job knowledge, and all the other vast body of information we carry around with us.

However, we have to put "permanent" into quotation marks because, actually, most of our long-term memories do fade over time. We knew a lot more about medieval history just before we passed the exam in college than we remember today. And we remember a great deal more about our current everyday lives than we remember about our lives of just a few years or even months ago. (You probably know the name of the current vice president of the United States, but try to remember quickly all the vice presidents who have served during your lifetime. Even if you can recall them at all, it will probably take you quite a few minutes.)

◆ **Remote Memory.** Finally, there is the essentially unforgettable knowledge, much of which seems to have been with us all our lives, that we shall always remember this side of Alzheimer's disease. This includes everything from knowing our own names and those of our long-time friends, to memories of our childhood, to how to recite "Humpty Dumpty." Even if, as a result of disease, we seem to have dropped part of this information from our conscious memory, it will come back to us very quickly with only a slight reminder. Thus, for example, if we are immigrants from Poland, we may not speak our native language for 40 years, only to shake off its dust and become fluent again after a mere couple of weeks in Warsaw.

Another example of remote memories coming back to the surface was first observed by the Canadian brain surgeon Wilder Penfield during his seminal 1950s work doing neurosurgery to relieve focal epilepsy. Dr. Penfield and his colleagues used an electric probe to stimulate parts of the cortex of alert patients preparing to undergo brain surgery. They found that they could often elicit apparently long-forgotten memories, both real ones and "generic" ones, i.e., "typical" scenes that were not precise memories.

It has been estimated that long-term memory can store

MEMORY MOMENT _____

> ⁶⁶**A** *man's real possession is his memory. In nothing else is he rich, in nothing else is he poor."*

—Alexander Smith,
nineteenth-century Scottish poet.

a quadrillion (10^{15}) bits of information during a lifetime in different regions of the brain. For instance, the sounds of language, the meaning of words, and the various sensory memories are all stored in different sites.

Remote memory is usually not in the forefront of our consciousness until we need to use it. As we wrote this book, sometimes we relied on facts we had learned in college but had not needed to remember or draw upon for a long time, yet they were there. Once we do need it, we transfer the information from our remote into our long-term memory, whence we can easily retrieve and use it. Failure to complete this transfer can result in an experience we have all had, the "tip-of-the-tongue" phenomenon. We "know" the word or fact we want, but cannot recall it. We may have some sense of the rhythm of the word, the number of syllables in it, or even, sometimes, words with which it rhymes, but we can't access the word itself. Only later, usually when we're least expecting it, will the word often slip unbidden into our conscious memory. This experience becomes more frequent and harder to overcome as we age.

Remote memory has one other interesting characteristic, namely that our preferences and feelings can be shaped by encounters and experiences lodged that we don't consciously remember at all. For example, exposure to negative words flashed too quickly on a screen for them to register in conscious awareness caused people later to feel hostility toward a fictional person. Participants had no sense that they were remembering any negative information. And, in another experiment, anesthetized patients given suggestions that they would make a quick recovery actually did spend less time in the hospital postoperatively than patients who were not given such suggestions. Yet none of the patients remembered the suggestions.[15] Remote memory is a rather tricky phenomenon!

The Ways Different Types of Memory Decline

These four types of memory—immediate, short-term, long-term, and remote—decline at different rates with advancing age. Thus, the degree to which age-related loss needs to be "cured" varies too.

The first and last types of memory, i.e., immediate and remote, decline relatively little. In the case of immediate memory, the phenomenon is hardly memory at all; it is merely the ability to reproduce, for a very short time, a simple piece of information that is perceived to have little or no lasting value. Even if our ability to remember such material declines drastically, say by 50 percent, that would only mean that, to remember what we immediately need, we would have to concentrate 50 percent more—a large percentage increase, but nevertheless an insignificant absolute increase. Perhaps we might have to glance at the phone number three times while we are dialing instead of once or twice. But as a practical matter, this would make little difference to us.

At the other end of the scale, remote memory (also known as procedural memory) is so deeply embedded that we do not forget what it contains. Our remote memories constitute the bedrock on which all our short- and long-term memories rest. It is therefore unlikely to dissipate, unless our minds have become so eroded from disease or damage that we can no longer remember anything at all. Even then, many of these basal memories persist. For example, an avid lifelong golfer who had sunk into the final throes of AD was taken to a golf course. He had no idea what day it was, where he was, by whom he was accompanied, or what game was being played. He certainly had no idea why he was there. Yet, when shown a golf bag, he chose an appropriate club, and his swing, while stiff and a bit ungainly, still showed hints of his former elegant style.

The main declines in memory, then, come at the short-term and long-term levels. Of these, the declines in short-term memory are the more apparent for two reasons. The first is that, because large segments of the long-term memory are so well established that they approach almost the quality of remote memory, they are highly resistant to being forgotten. Thus, only a portion of long-term memory, i.e., that part adjunctive to the short-term, is easily subject to age-related decline.

The second reason that short-term memory declines are more apparent than long-term declines is that they carry with them more observable symptoms of memory shortcomings. With a declining short-term memory, the ability to remember names, faces, appointments, to commit a speech or a poem to memory, or to recall where we put our keys, all decline—and that decline is very noticeable both to the people forgetting and to their family and friends.

Fortunately, as we shall show in a later chapter, short-term memory is also the area most conducive to improvement by mind exercises. Thus, for example, actors who are used to memorizing lines—initially an act of short-term memory, although it may turn into long-term memory if the play succeeds or the actor cares enough—can continue to achieve prodigious memorization feats well into old age.

BY CONTENT

If memory can be categorized by its duration, it can also be viewed from an entirely different perspective, namely by type of content. Of course this breakdown could splinter the quality of remembering into a thousand subcategories. There is no end to the types of things you remember. However, for our purposes, it will be sufficient to differentiate just three: facts (called episodic memory by many experts); knowledge (often called semantic memory); and procedural memory. Let us examine the meaning of memory from these perspectives.

◆ **Events and Facts.** Factual memory is entirely straightforward: it is the ability to remember individual bits of information. It includes everything from remembering that one and one makes two, to recalling the name of the President of the United States. It also includes the memory of specific events which define much of what we experience in life: high school graduations, birthdays, weddings, funerals, and, of course, all the personal traumas and joys of our lives. Individual facts and events are the most easily forgotten of all types of memory—the more easily, the more isolated they are. Thus, new facts that come to our attention in context with our existing body of knowledge are relatively easy to assimilate and remember, whereas facts that are unrelated to other facts we already know are more easily forgotten. For example, if a new study on memory were to be published tomorrow in the *New England Journal of Medicine,* both of us would quickly learn and remember any new facts it provided. However, if we happen to notice that, in the adjacent *Journal* article, new information was presented about the tensile strength of babies' knee tendons, we would probably not remember that at all.

The act of relating facts we want to learn—or want to remember—to a preexisting body of information we already own is the basis for improving our factual memory. As we shall explain in more detail in a later chapter, most techniques for improving memory (by which is most often meant improving the memory of facts) boil down to developing ways of positioning the new facts to be remembered into a pattern of already known information.

◆ **Knowledge.** Knowledge, and the memory that underlies it, is different from memory for events and facts. What we understand—whether it be the ability to speak one or more languages, the know-how to do mental arithmetic, the capability to sing a recognizable tune, or the capacity to write a book on memory—obviously involves our knowing many related facts. But this is only part of the story. For knowledge is much more subtle than merely the accumulation of facts. Assuming that we could memorize the meaning of every single word in the *Oxford English Dictionary,* if we did not actually speak English we would still have a great deal of trouble making ourselves understood. Thus, knowledge is really a synthesis of an immeasurably large body of facts until their sum melds into a memory amalgam that gives us insight, judgment, and hopefully even wisdom. Often we call this immeasurably large group of individually unrecalled memories *experience.*

One example of the benefits of greater knowledge, which seems like a better memory, is that older adults perform remarkably better than younger adults in telling family stories, especially those related to their own past. In this way, older people help prevent what Dr. D. L. Schacter calls "cultural amnesia." Not only do older adults constitute a living legacy for their own families, but throughout time it is the elders who have kept the lore, the historical adventures, and the momentous events of their community or culture alive for the enjoyment of succeeding generations. "When older adults were asked to tell some personal stories from anytime in their past," Dr. Schacter writes, "raters who read the narratives judged the elderly's stories to be of higher quality—more engaging and dramatic—than those of the young."[16]

Generally, knowledge is more resistant to forgetfulness than are facts. This is simply because knowledge is made up of so many facts that it is unlikely that they will all be forgotten at the same time. Consequently, the remembered ones provide the context for those that might otherwise drop from memory. In other words, knowledge is less easily forgotten than individual facts because its information is so tightly woven together that none of it can easily "slip through the cracks."

The problem with knowledge, of course, is that, while it is not easily forgotten, it is also not easily gained. Thus, at any age, assimilating new knowledge—taking a new course at college, mastering a new skill, learning about a new neighborhood—takes time and trouble. The good news is that, while it may require effort, learning new knowledge is not only possible but very practical at any age. Moreover, while it may take an older person longer than a younger one to internalize new knowledge, once the effort is made and the knowledge assimilated into long-term memory, it will not be easily lost.

Thus, here again is a very useful way not to suffer an unacceptable decline in memory as we age. Sure, we may forget more. But in spite of that, if we keep on learning, we may end up in old age with a larger pile of remembered knowledge than we had when we were young. We may even become the beneficiary of the rather jealous praise, "She's forgotten more than I ever knew!"

◆ **Procedural Memory.** This is the most basic type of memory of all. It is the memory of how we move, and act, and "have our being." As stated earlier, procedural memories are not often forgotten or even reduced except at the extremes of a mind-destroying disease. Until the day that we die we shall remember how to walk, pick up our glass and drink, drive a car, ride a bicycle, or sign our names. Of course, physical debility may prevent these activities; but, in the absence of serious brain disease, if we can't walk, it's a muscular or skeletal problem, not a mental one.

HOW MEMORIES ARE FORMED

The final step in understanding what we need to know about memory in order to learn how to avoid its decline with age deals with understanding how memories are formed in the first place. This is important because the quality of our overall memories depends on two factors: what we remember, or fail to forget, thus storing up previously known facts; and what we learn fresh, or relearn at the point of forgetting, thus adding to our store of factual information. To oversimplify, it is probably fair to say that, if the sum of what we remember and/or learn is as great as the sum of what we forget, then for practical purposes our memory has improved even though our ability to remember new data may be slower, and our tendency to lose old data greater. And if we gain more facts than we lose, would it not be fair to say that our memory has improved? After all, in that case we have access to more usable stored information. That it required more effort to maintain this quantity of facts, and that it has become more difficult to assimilate new ones, is also true. But that is a separate issue. The happy state of affairs that pertains is that we now remember as many or more facts than we did previously. That, surely, is what *effective* memory is all about.

There are four processes, or memory generators, that can cause us to forget, misremember, or remember something:

◆ **Paying Attention.** This is probably the single most important aspect of gathering new, memorable information. We shall discuss this subject in more detail later, but for now suffice it to state the obvious, namely, that you'll never remember anything to which you paid no attention initially. Thus, you will notice the houses on either side of the street as you drive by them, but you will pay them no heed, and remember nothing about them the moment you are past. Even if you concentrate on some object briefly, such as the cars surrounding you, your concentration is only on a single, temporary plane—to make sure that you don't have a collision. You take no note of the cars in other ways, and therefore forget everything about them the moment they are out of harm's way.

Less obviously, people who have trouble remembering the names of the folk to whom they are introduced weren't paying attention in the first place, when the introductions were made. We can rectify this forgetfulness through inattention (which is not actually forgetting but rather never assimilating the information in the first place) by making a conscious effort to pay attention.

We are less likely to forget topics or information that we are interested in than things that are not important to us. Anita Loos, author of *Gentlemen Prefer Blondes,* knew this when she wrote "Gentlemen always seem to remember blondes." And noted memory expert K. L. Higbee recounts the following story to illustrate the same point:

> A returning serviceman is met at the airport by his girlfriend. As an attractive stewardess walks by, he says to her, "That's Laura Nelson."
>
> "How do you know?" asks the girlfriend.
>
> "Oh, the names of all the crew members were posted at the front of the plane," he casually replies.
>
> He couldn't answer her next question: "What was the pilot's name?"[17]

◆ **Selectivity.** One of the advantages of growing older is that we are likely to have a better handle on what is important and what is not. As noted, paying attention is the first key to remembering. But, obviously, we don't want to (and can't) pay attention to everything. Therefore, selectivity is the key to remembering the "right" things, i.e., those that are important to our lives.

We have often heard the remark "She has a selective memory" used pejoratively. And, of course, remembering only bad things about a person can be destructive behavior. However, innately, selective memory is a powerful tool for holding onto or even improving memory—or more specifically *effective* memory—with age. A brilliant acquaintance used to turn off his hearing aid when someone prattled on at him about nothing much, the while smiling benignly and occasionally nodding his head in agreement. "Why waste my finite mental capacity on rubbish," he would demand, "when I could be listening to Mozart in my head or recalling a Shakespeare sonnet in my mind's eye?" Learning how to sift out what is important from what is not is one of the memory-enhancing techniques we'll discuss more fully later.

Another form of selectivity is what our brains do for us, without our fully realizing, when they filter out and eliminate interfering noises and sights before we even become aware of them—or, if we are aware, before they can disrupt us too much.

Sandy moved to downtown San Francisco, where the sirens of emergency vehicles are never silent, day or night. She quickly learned not to hear them, unless she was on the street where it made a difference. Consequently, she was quite surprised when her mother visited and after the first night complained that the sirens had kept her awake all night. By the end of two weeks, her mother was sleeping through the night also.

◆ **Adaptive Remembering and Forgetting.** This is somewhat akin to selectivity, except that it is largely, and often entirely, unconscious. We forget those things which it would hurt us to remember, and remember those things it would hurt us to forget. For example, the trauma of childbirth is something most women forget. If they did not, they might be too fearful of the remembered pain to have another child. Conversely, they usually remember the rush of joy they felt the first time they saw or cuddled or breast-fed their newborn. That's what "makes it all worthwhile."

This tendency to adapt our memories so that they do not hurt us explains why the memory of emotionally traumatic events, even where they are preserved for a lifetime, are often distorted. Psychiatrist Lenore Terr's studies of the 26 children kidnapped at gunpoint on a school bus in Chowchilla, California, show this effect. When Dr. Terr interviewed 23 of the children four to five years after the event, she found a number of rather striking errors and distortions. She believes that these developed not only as a result of perceptual errors at the time of the event, but were also caused by the later unconscious effort to mitigate the stress of the memory of the terrifying episode. Seven of eight children, whose memories were accurate when questioned in an interview shortly after the kidnapping, exhibited distortions during the later interviewing. For example, one child remembered a pair of female kidnappers (there were none) in addition to the male kidnappers. Another remembered that one of the kidnappers had pillows stuffed in his pants, also a mistaken memory.[18]

While adaptive memory is often unconscious, it can also be consciously influenced. You can practice forgetting the bad things that happen to you and, with conscious effort, replace them with memories of the good times. After all, if you are concentrating hard on remembering and visualizing the day you won the contest, you cannot concurrently be depressed by the memory of how badly you did the year before.

Indeed, many cases of clinical depression can be explained as the malfunction of adaptive memory: depressed people remember the things that are bad for them to remember. While it would be naive to suggest that all depression can be cured by an act of will, i.e., by remembering the good times and banishing the memory of the bad, there is a sound basis to cognitive therapy and other psychological approaches that use this method as a key weapon in their arsenal of techniques for treating depression.

More practically, there is little doubt that a bad mood—a sort of limited or temporary depression—will also give rise to maladaptive memory retention, albeit in comparatively minor degree. Whereas making a conscious effort to banish depression may be impossible for most depressed people, banishing or at least mitigating a dark mood is a lot more feasible. In so doing, you will be concentrating on remembering the good times. As a result (since they are more fun to remember), you will probably find your memory improving. At the very least, you will *feel* as if it is improving. Therefore, you will have the sense of well-being that accompanies improved memory, and you will "feel better about yourself." Your memory will either improve, or, at worst, you will be as happy as if it had!

◆ **Misremembering.** Part of the complexity in determining exactly how and why we forget as we age stems first from the basic fact that human memory is imperfect at all ages. Memories are not exact recordings of an experience. To some extent we use our knowledge of the world and similar experiences to "fill in" incomplete or missing information in our memories. These "gap fillers" may be valid, but they can just as easily lead to memory error, which, when called to our attention, may seem like memory loss.

Recent theories of how the brain works influence the whole question of whether memories are "true" or "false." A large body of research has shown that memories are often somewhat distorted. Indeed, as any historian will tell you, past events can be interpreted in many different ways with no one set of recollections representing the absolute "truth." Recovered memories may be particularly unreliable, especially in borderline patients who may have had a distorted perception of the interpersonal events to begin with.[19] According to the research of Nobel prize–winning neuroscientist Dr. Gerald Edelman, the brain chooses images, sounds, and other sensations and interpretations registered in the past and then combines them to produce what we call a memory. This "memory" may be an accurate depiction of something that happened, but it can just as easily be a personal creation, using information from various incidents.[20]

It's very likely that in trauma, when emotions and sensations are intense—and may even be on overload—that the actual memory of the experience is fragmented. Consequently, only fragments of a remembered traumatic event are likely to be entirely accurate when they are re-remembered, while other parts may be derived from different experiences as the aroused nervous system searches around and tries to comprehend the re-aroused emotion.

Cognitive psychologist Craig Barclay asked college students to keep a diary in which they recorded things that happened to them just after they occurred (actual memories). Dr. Barclay collected the diaries and subsequently tested the students' memories for these events at delays ranging from several months to two years. Sometimes he showed them a printed version of an actual diary and asked them if this was exactly what they had written down. Other times the descriptions were changed in various respects, like adding that a person had hunted for a gift in ten stores before giving up, when, in fact, she had never written that in her diary. As time passed, students increasingly agreed that the changed descriptions (false memories) were exactly what they had written down earlier.[21]

Naturally, then, as people age, more and more false memories of long past events will occur. While this does not mean that, in theory, older people's memories of immediate facts will necessarily be worse, it does suggest that older people's memories may be more confused by incorrectly remembered data. Therefore, they are more likely to confuse all memory, distant or fairly recent. (For example, if you incorrectly remember that San Diego is north of San Francisco, you will probably also misre-member its climatic conditions. Your current memory will be confused by incorrect earlier information.)

What Type of AAMI Needs to Be Cured?

Once we understand that immediate and remote memory does not degrade significantly, that knowledge only fades very slowly, and that procedural memory hardly declines at all, we know where we need to concentrate our memory-improving efforts. Short- and long-term memory (and especially where the two approach one another, i.e., lengthy short- and short-duration long-term memory) are where we need to work. And those efforts should be aimed at learning how to hold onto factual information by fitting it into a pattern of the rest of our less fragile, more permanent matrix of memories.

Retrieval versus Recall

One final matter, before we move on, about what constitutes memory and what we should do about it: Remembered facts are only useful to the extent that they are available to us when we need them. Therefore, not only do we have to be able to store information in our memories, but we also have to be able to retrieve it at will and reasonably quickly. Unfortunately, that retrieval mechanism slows down with age, which is a major reason we think that our memories are weakening.

There are three main reasons why retrieval slows:

◆ One of the most important is that we simply have too many facts from which to choose. This is, of course, where selectivity comes into play as the

MEMORY MOMENT _____

RETRIEVING MEMORIES

R etrieval *means remembering something we once knew. One word from the prompter usually causes the actor to remember the entire monologue.*

Recall, *a more active kind of retrieval, involves a deliberate self-initiated search to remember something that is not in the present ("What are the state capitals?"). Recall is more difficult than recognition, which is why it is harder to remember names than to remember faces. When we say "I can't remember," we usually mean "I can't recall."*

method of eliminating the unessential and so making essential memories more easily unearthed.

◆ We concentrate less intensely on finding the information we seek as we get older. "Oh, it'll come to me," we think and move on to the next subject. This may be useful adaptive behavior, provided that we do not permit it to escalate into the sort of mental laziness that will certainly interfere with our thinking processes including our memories.

◆ And, most importantly, the speed with which we can retrieve information slows because, as we shall describe, the conductivity of our brains decreases as we age, hence the speed and accuracy of the electrically coded messages that carry memory declines. This problem is chemically induced and therefore, thankfully, can be chemically cured.

Summary: What Is Memory?

While memory is, obviously, the ability to remember all matters, the part that is most prone to decline—and on which we must therefore concentrate—is the short- to medium-term memory of facts. These memories have been created and more or less finely honed, and can therefore be re-created and strengthened by: paying attention to what is to be remembered; sifting out those matters which are worth remembering; anchoring them into a preexistent matrix of well-remembered data; and, as far as possible, concentrating on those memories that are "good for us."

2

Why Do We Forget?

The chemical aging of our cells

♦

Fighting off the memory busters

♦

Becoming rusty with disuse

♦

Poor health, the wrong food (and too much of it), and the wrong nutritional supplements

♦

Stress: Look at it as fun

♦

Beat the blues

♦

I.Q. and education make a difference

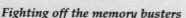

What's going on here?

Why exactly does memory, especially short-term memory and the long-term memory adjacent to it, decline with age? What are the inner and outer influences that cause memory to degrade?

To provide you with a clear understanding of just why

your capacity to remember tends to decline with age, let us first list the six main reasons. Then, in the balance of this chapter, we shall briefly expand upon each of them. Those expanded descriptions will then provide the foundation on which, in chapters 3 and 4, we shall provide you with solutions.

Remember, as you read the following list, in spite of all those reasons your memory declines, it doesn't have to. We now know how to delay, avoid, or even largely reverse age-associated memory impairment (AAMI).

THE SIX REASONS FOR AAMI

There are six basic reasons that, left unattended, our memories weaken with age:

1 The conductivity of our cells, i.e., their ability to carry the electrical messages that generate memory, declines with age as a result of chemical and structural changes in the brain.

2 Outside influences interfere with our memories, dimming, confusing, rearranging, or even blocking them. These influences include perceptual problems we may develop with age such as reduced hearing or seeing acuity. While these do not directly interfere with memory, they reduce our gaining full control of what is to be remembered.

 MEMORY MOMENT _____

We might all feel happier if we could agree with the renowned American writer and publisher E. G. Hubbard, who said, "A retentive memory is a good thing, but the ability to forget is the true token of greatness."

3 As a result of those two factors, we find it harder to add new information to our data bank and therefore are less motivated to do so, leaving our memories to become "rusty" from disuse.

4 Too often, we eat a poor diet, augmented by the wrong boosting nutritional supplements (or none at all), exercise too little, possibly drink too much alcohol and/or smoke, and thus become overweight, sluggish, and prone to poor health, low energy, and actual diseases. Naturally this overall poor health worsens our memories as it worsens all our mental and physical functions.

5 Stress, a constant in most of our lives, adversely affects memory.

6 Depression heightens our sense that our memories are failing far more quickly than they really are. This fear adds even more stress and lowers our motivation to fight our real memory declines (because to do so seems "hopeless"), thus converting our misevaluation into a self-fulfilling prophecy.

As we shall prove in the balance of this book, each of these six factors can be fought, delayed, and largely overcome by our Memory Maximization program. Let us, therefore, examine each of them in a little more depth to understand their genesis and negative impact and so prepare ourselves to overcome them.

The Chemical Aging of Our Cells

As we have said, memory isn't a "thing," nor is there one place in our brains that we can pinpoint as the "seat of memory." Rather, memory is a vastly complicated and convoluted network of electrochemical conductors and electrical impulses. While each of those individual impulses is transitory, their traces remain as a pattern. It is that pattern that constitutes what we remember. And it is the ease with which we form new patterns that defines how well we are able to assimilate and retain new information.

It all begins in the brain and spinal cord, and their most basic unit, the nerve cell or *neuron*. The brain contains about 100 billion neurons plus twice as many cells (called neuroglia or just *glia*) that provide structural and metabolic support for the neurons. Each neuron is a link in a complicated network of neuronal pathways that provide thousands of connections with other neurons.

Although our entire bodies are composed of cells, neurons are distinguished from other cells in that they specialize in conducting chemical and electrical impulses. It is the flow of these currents that determines our thought processes.

Unlike many other cells, brain cells have great sensitivity to oxygen deprivation. Neurons die within a few minutes if they do not receive oxygen. Although brain cells are designed to live a long time, once a brain cell dies or is damaged, it generally cannot be replaced, although new evidence is accumulating that indicates that sometimes, under the right conditions, this is not true and the brain can and does grow new cells. Nevertheless, as a rule, the older you are the fewer brain cells you have available. In itself, this reduction is not critical, but it could become so if the remaining cells also function less efficiently than they needed to (or did) previously. Therefore, to prevent their own death, living neurons constantly must maintain themselves. If cell cleanup and repair slows down, as it may as we age, the neurons cannot function at full efficiency.

MEMORY MOMENT

> *The scientific study of memory began in the early 1870s when a German philosopher, Hermann Ebbinghaus, broke with a two-thousand-year-old tradition that held that memory was the province of the philosopher and not of scientists.*

There are several different types of neurons in the brain, which affect different parts of the body. For instance, a motor neuron transmits energy impulses to muscles to "tell" them to move, or to glands to activate them to secrete hormones. Sensory neurons transmit sensory impulses. They give us information about what we see, hear, feel, taste, and smell; hence, they are the original source of most of our memories (although a few memories do originate from imagination or dreams).

Neurons are surrounded by a cell membrane and have gossamer-thin fibers or filaments extending from them

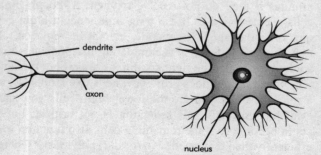

Fig. 2.1: **The Neuron**

Neurons, the most basic unit of the brain, conduct electrical and chemical impulses. The dendrites look like antennae and pass impulses to the neuron's center, the nucleus.

which transmit signals from one neuron to another. A typical neuron has a cell body with a dark, central nucleolus. Projecting from one edge of the cell body are many *dendrites,* part of the neuron's filamentous network (see Fig. 2.1).

Acting like antennae, dendrites receive impulses from other neurons and conduct them along to the cell's center. They are like the branches of a tree, relatively thick as they emerge from the cell, but dividing often and becoming thinner at each branch point (a configuration called "arborization"). Unfortunately dendrites are very fragile and easily damaged, especially by aging, so that they gradually become less effective at receiving and conducting impulses. The good news is that research with rats has shown that this aging-induced loss of these branching "spines" can be partly avoided. The even better news is that researchers have found that dendrites can grow new protrusions or spines in response to new experiences. In other words, exercising the mind (one of the key parts of our Memory Maximizing plan) actually improves our physical capacity for memory.

Extending from one end of the neuron is a larger single *axon,* which conducts nerve impulses to the dendrites of other neurons. It is possible for an axon to extend 1 meter (3.3 feet) or more. Glia or supporting cells wrap around axons to form an insulating layer or membrane called *myelin,* or the myelin sheath. Myelin helps to reduce the loss of electrical current from the axon.

Each axon and dendrite has many tiny branches that connect it to other neurons, so that a single neuron can communicate with thousands of others. The specialized point of contact between the axon of one neuron and the dendrites of another is an infinitesimal space called the *synapse.* A single neuron can have as many as 100,000 synapses connecting it with other neurons (see Fig. 2.2).

"Messages"—really electrical nerve impulses—travel down the axon until they reach the synapse, where they cause the release, from the end of the axon, of "little packets" of chemicals, called neurotransmitters. Nerve cells and their neurotransmitters work very fast. It takes no more than one-thousandth of a second for a neuron to send the electrical signal that it has fired, or activated, to the end of the axon. As the neurotransmitter crosses the ultra-microscopic synaptic space and reaches the dendrites of the next neuron, it activates specific receptors, sensitive proteins, embedded in the receiving cell's membranes. As between a lock and key, the connection or "binding" is highly specific. Each neurotransmitter recognizes and "grabs hold" of only a specific type of receptor. In this way—miraculously, it seems to many of us—thoughts are conveyed throughout our brains until they reach the activating point from which new signals

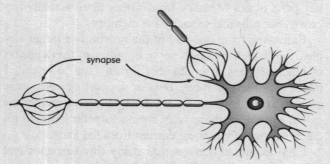

Fig. 2.2: The Synapse

To communicate, the axon of one neuron passes the impulse to the dendrites of another. This infinitesimal point of contact is called the synapse.

cause us to do something about them (or, perhaps, think new thoughts). Those thoughts, and the actions they generate, are usually soon over and done with. But the pathways they followed, especially if they are used repeatedly, remain and become one bit of our memory.

THE NEED FOR PHOSPHOLIPIDS IN CELL MEMBRANES

Lying next to the receptors, and making up the bulk of the membrane of each cell, are molecules of *phospholipids,* with which the receptors have chemical bonds. Even though there are other lipids and protein compounds in the membranes, phospholipids make up as much as 70% of the membrane's structural components.[22] The nutritional supplement at the heart of this book is a phospholipid. Its function is to help activate and regulate many of the membranes' proteins. Simply stated, adding to your phospholipid supply by daily taking the supplement we shall recommend solves many of the problems that lead to age-associated memory impairment.

Once a transmitter has attached to, or "bound" with, its receptor, a cascade of biochemical interactions are triggered that relay the message to the neuron's central cell body, whence it progresses to the end of the new cell's axon, where it continues the same process of passing the message to other cells by releasing its own transmitters. One Italian researcher summarized it this way: In order to trigger an appropriate or adequate response in the cell, the biochemical messages that reach the neuronal surface must be "captured, recognized, decodified, transformed, and relayed in the proper form to the inside of the cell."[23]

To put the whole picture into perspective: a piece of brain the size of a grain of rice contains 1 million nerve cells, 10 billion synapses, and 20 miles of axons. Each of these nerve cells both "hears from" and "talks to" as many as 10,000 other cells.[24] Millions of signals flash through the brain all the time. Researchers have learned to see the locations of other neurons with which an individual nerve cell connects by injecting a colored dye into the cell, enabling them to piece together a "map" of brain cell connections.[25] These maps show clearly that older brains have fewer "points of contact" than younger ones, and this decline is where we need to concentrate our efforts if we are to maintain our memories at the same level of efficiency as in our youth.

One reason that our brains are susceptible to short-

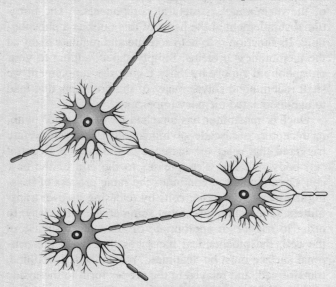

Fig. 2.3: Mapping the Brain

To preserve memory, the connections between the billions of neurons in your brain are vital. Scans have revealed that older brains have fewer of these connections.

term memory loss is that, as we enter the decades of our sixties and seventies, they lose density, their circuits becoming thinned out. Consequently, their blood flow, uptake of oxygen, and utilization of glucose (sugar) decreases significantly. Research on memory tasks that involve processes in the frontal lobe shows that they are especially affected by these aging processes.[26] Low blood sugar, or inability to use the sugar that is available, causes the brain—and especially the hippocampus—to have an energy shortage analogous to an electrical blackout which reduces some forms of short-term memory.

THE SWITCHBOARD OF MEMORY

As we explained earlier, neurons produce chemical signals and electrical messages that jump across the synapses between our brain cells, and memories are stored, not in the neurons or synapses themselves, but rather in the *pattern* of connections between neurons. Initial memory storage involves changes in the strength of those patterns. In other words, when a new piece of information comes along, it embeds itself in our memory by changing the pattern of the electrical impulses that transport that new piece of information through our neurons. Long-term memory storage, therefore, involves the growth of new synaptic connections between neurons.

As we age, neurons and their synapses, especially those passing through channels of neurons which are not in constant use, tend to become less conductive to electrical impulses. In effect, unused channels or patterns become "closed" or even disappear—much as a disused waterway might silt up and become unnavigable—thus fading or entirely wiping out little-used memories. Only the main channels of our minds, the ones we use constantly, remain as open as ever.

It follows that, if we can improve the conductivity of the highly fragile and complicated neuron/synapse cellular system we have described, we will have solved the first, basic piece of the puzzle of how to minimize, avoid, or even reverse AAMI. That is what the nutritional supplement described in the next chapter will do.

For simplicity's sake, we described the action of a single impulse in sending its electrical and chemical "messages." In fact, however, every nerve and neuronal pathway is made up of many bundles, which in turn are made up of hundreds and hundreds of axons. Together the nervous tissue of the brain (its outer layer or cortex) and the spinal cord make up "the little gray cells" that author Agatha Christie's famed detective hero Hercule Poirot is so fond of using to best Scotland Yard in solving crime—the implication being that the Yard detectives act before thinking. Actually the cells are more tan than gray, but can you ever imagine Poirot pointing to his head and saying with his inimitable Belgian accent, "the little tan cells at work"?

Thus, the first reason for AAMI is the gradual reduction in the electrical conductivity of our cells. We can fight back by taking the appropriate phospholipid as a nutritional supplement.

  MEMORY MOMENT _____

> **66** **T**he Right Honourable gentleman is indebted
> to his memory for his jests, and to his
> imagination for his facts."
>
> —Richard Brinsley Sheridan,
> during a speech in the
> British House of Commons
> replying to the remarks
> of a Mr. Dundas.

Fighting Off the Memory Busters

A common belief is that we forget because new and old memories get in each other's way and "crowd" our brain. "My mind is too cluttered," said one elderly woman. "I simply have too much stuff in there to remember it all."

Possibly it is true that the myriad of inconsequential topics we encountered in the past get pushed out by the newer trivia of today. But, in general, the more information you learn, or store, about a specific subject, or subjects, the more you aid your ability to remember: that past knowledge makes it easier both to understand and to learn the new information about the same subject. Familiarity makes it easier to organize information in order to learn and retain it.[27] Then what is it, apart from your changing brain chemistry, that causes you to forget?

There are any number of outside forces that interfere with our ability, and even with our desire, to fully exercise our memories. Among the most important—or perhaps pernicious—of these are:

◆ **Inattention.** As we have stated previously, inattention is a main reason for "forgetting" or, more properly, for not learning. Clearly, we must learn something before we can remember it, and to do this we must pay attention to the material we are learning. If you're supposed to learn something that is not very interesting or important to you, you may not work at it very hard, and you are not likely to remember it as well as you would remember information that is highly interesting or meaningful to you. Older persons sometimes have trouble paying attention because they "have heard it all before" (even though they have forgotten) and are too bored to bother to relearn it.

◆ **Discarding Unwanted Memories.** A major proponent of the belief that we can willfully "lose" memories—and often do so as we age—is the well-known neuroscientist Larry S. Squire. Dr. Squire reminds us that, since the formation and use of memory is a dynamic process, the content of memory will change as interfering information is acquired and affects preexisting memory. "New information-storage episodes constantly occur," says Dr. Squire, "resculpturing previously existing representations . . . and changing the structure of memory."[28] Moreover, as Dr. Squire emphasizes, the truth is that we don't want to remember everything that has ever happened to us and, in that sense, forgetting is an adaptive and "economical response to the demands placed on memory by the environment in which we live."[29] According to Dr. Squire, the fact that certain cues or reminders can elicit the recall of typically unavailable memories demonstrates that the brain stores more memories than we use regularly, but also suggests that, if they are not recalled ("used") over a certain period, they will be discarded. He agrees with most other researchers that there is no evidence that all past experiences are permanently represented.

◆ **Disuse.** Decay is a shorthand term for the idea that, if a particular memory is not used often, as may happen as people age, the neuronal connections or pathways between the nerve cells weaken and eventually the memory is lost through lack of regular use.

Experiments with cats and monkeys show this clearly. When one eye is kept covered while they are young, the neuronal connections served by that eye are weakened. If the side of eye closure is switched early enough, the neural connectivity related to knowledge is regained, but a similar loss then occurs in the newly deprived eye and visual cortext. This suggests that new experiences affect the nervous system by directly strengthening or weakening synaptic connections.[30]

What that means, of course, is that we can impact what we remember—and what we forget—by exercising our minds and "going over" or reviewing the information we want to be able to recall. Often this involves no more than seeking out some touchstone to unleash prior memories, much as a photo of an almost forgotten event brings back lively memories of the whole event itself.

A specific example of such memory triggers is olfactory memory because many of our earliest childhood memories are of smell. In Proust's great novel *Remembrance of Things Past,* he describes how the taste and smell of a madeleine cake soaked in lime tea like the one his aunt Léonie used to give him on Sunday mornings brought back a number of vivid memories of his childhood: the old gray house where his aunt lived, the town where the house was located, the town square and various streets in the town, even the country roads around the town where they used to travel when the weather was good.

No doubt, you have similar taste and smell memories of your own that segue into a host of other memories. The memory of a grandmother's fragrance as she picked you up. The smell of baked goods or a freshly mowed lawn. We know a woman who tries in vain with various commercial products she puts in her apartment dryer to

❖ MEMORY MOMENT _____

> 66 **E** ducation is what you have left over after you have forgotten everything you have learned."
> —Old adage.

get the fragrance of sun-dried clothes. She loves to visit friends in the country who still use an outdoor clothesline so that she can sleep between sheets that bring back all sorts of childhood memories. A recent study showed that about 85 percent of people have a childhood memory linked to a particular aroma and that memories triggered by an odor tend to be more emotionally intense and evocative than those linked to other cues.[31] It's understandable, then, that olfactory memories are some of our most pleasant ones.

Dr. Alan Hirsch, a neurologist and psychiatrist at the Smell and Taste Treatment and Research foundation in Chicago, is investigating the impact odors can have on learning and memory. After testing a variety of fragrances that had no effect (lavender, jasmine, the smell of baked goods), he finally found a mixed floral fragrance that he claims more than doubles the speed of learning compared to a no-odor condition.[32]

He believes that we'll eventually scent our classrooms and offices to accelerate learning and use aromas to speed up rehabilitation for people who've had strokes or brain injuries.

◆ **Interference from Material Learned** *After* **the Memory.** One of the newest pieces of information about remembering and forgetting was announced recently when scientists at Johns Hopkins University reported that

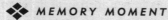

❖ MEMORY MOMENT

D r. Hirsch discovered that when teachers administered a word list in the presence of a butterscotch or peppermint smell, and then introduced the smells once again when the children were asked to remember the lists, their memory improved.

we have a six-hour "window of vulnerability" in learning new motor or performance skills. Researchers Reza Shadmehr and Henry H. Holcomb say it takes that long for the brain to consolidate all of the neural pathways that control the task and if a person tries to learn another new performance skill during this time, the previous learning may slip from memory.[33] This "trumping" of a prior memory is called "retroactive inhibition," and refers to the forgetting of older material because of "interference" from similar new material.

As described above, retroactive inhibition normally occurs within six hours of the original acquisition of the material to be learned. For instance, Bill's wife called him at the office and asked him to pick up a few things at the supermarket on his way home. Bill, who prided himself on his memory skill, wrote the list down, read it through again before he left the office, and casually tossed the list into the trash. As he left the office, his secretary went over with him a list of several important appointments he had the next day. When Bill got to the supermarket, he was embarrassed that he couldn't remember most of the items his wife had asked him to buy. In fact, if Bill had known a little more about his memory processes, he would have realized that his secretary's list of appointments had interfered with his earlier memory. A smarter Bill would have turned around and headed toward the trash can.

However, retroactive inhibition is not always limited to this circumstance, where new memory displaces old only when it follows closely on its heels. The phenomenon may also appear when the new memory, although much later in time than the old, is very similar to it. Naturally, as we age, the increased number of new memories we amass are increasingly likely to obliterate older mem-

MEMORY MOMENT _____

> J ohn Dean came to be known as the "man with
> the tape recorder memory" because he testified in
> such detail during the Watergate hearings about
> "remembered" conversations with Richard Nixon. The
> actual tapes of those conversations, however, show that
> his memory was only moderately accurate and
> sometimes quite inaccurate.

ories. How many of the names of your first-grade classmates can you remember? Probably very few because you had little reason to, and didn't keep using that list of names over the years. Instead you learned the names of other classmates as they came and went in your life.

◆ **Interference from Material Learned *Before* the Memory.** This is called "proactive inhibition." Have you ever had the experience of changing your phone number and then not being able to remember the new number? Or writing the wrong year on the first few checks in January? The old telephone number and last year's date were interfering with your memory of the new numbers.

◆ **False Information.** Noted researcher Elizabeth Loftus demonstrated in her classic studies on eyewitness memory that the memories of witnesses can be shaped by false information received after the event. In a series of experiments, Dr. Loftus showed a filmstrip of an accident. With one group of participants, she asked if another car passed the red car while it was at a stop sign (the truth). For a second group she asked if the car was passed while it was at a yield sign. When Dr. Loftus later asked people to describe the accident scene, more than 80 percent of those in the group where she had mentioned the yield sign remembered it as being in the scene.

MEMORY MOMENT _____

> 6 6 *It isn't so astonishing, the number of things I can remember, as the number of things I can remember that aren't so."*
>
> —Mark Twain.

Again, when discussing the accident with one group of filmstrip observers, Dr. Loftus referred to the cars as "smashing" into each other, while she used the term "hit each other" with other observers. A week later she asked if there had been broken glass at the scene (there had not). Only 14 percent of those with whom she had used the word "hit" thought there was glass, contrasted to 32 percent of the people who heard her say "smashed."[34] In similar fashion, police, interviewers, and reporters may deliberately, or unwittingly, influence eyewitness memory.

Such false memories are common to all age groups, but tend to be more pronounced among older people. This may be because initial attention is lower or partially impaired, or it may be a phenomenon of aging itself.

◆ **Absentmindedness.** This phenomenon, often associated with aging, is really just another form of failure to pay attention—although if it is repeated often enough, as with the caricature of the absent-minded professor, it feels as if it is a discrete "memory interferer." In fact, it is only that we are so busy thinking about what we are going to do at a business meeting, or about the many purchases we have to make while shopping, that we fail to pay attention to where we parked. When we come back to find the car, we haven't actually *forgotten* where we parked, we just didn't pay sufficient attention to where we were parking in the first place.[35] In general, high levels of anxiety tend to narrow our focus of attention onto important matters (the meeting), but away from unimportant ones (where we parked).

◆ **Prejudices and Beliefs.** Our preconceptions, particularly those that are culturally induced, often distort our memories. Two groups of students, one Spanish and the other English (48 in each group), successively observed two films showing events specific to Spain (a *romeria* or pilgrimage) and to England (a village fete) before participating in two kinds of memory tests: giving free recall and answering a verbal recognition test that contained "lures" consistent and inconsistent with cultural expectations. Half the subjects were instructed to adopt the role of an observer, while the remainder played the role of a participant. In a surprising turn, recall accuracy was greater for the event that was not from the person's own country, while recall errors were greater for the event from the person's own country. Recognition accuracy was higher for the event from the person's own country.[36]

◆ **Heightened Emotion.** A number of studies have shown that the greater the amount of emotion experienced by a witness to a crime, the less completely the witness will remember the events of the crime, with the memory of the central event being stronger, but that of the peripheral details being weaker.

Thus, the second reason for AAMI is that outside influences interfere with memory. The solution is to

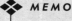 **MEMORY MOMENT** _____

    66A good storyteller is a person who has a good
      memory, and hopes other people haven't."
                            —Irvin S. Cobb, American humorist.

*concentrate harder—and do exercises to assist our con-
centration—on those things we really want to remember.*

Becoming Rusty with Disuse

Have you ever come home after a hard day, flopped
down in front of the television, and allowed yourself to
turn into a classic couch potato? Most of us have. Probably we realize that we would be better off reading that
new book the *New York Times* described as a "cogently
reasoned, thought-provoking, challenging" seven-hun-
dred-page "masterpiece." But we just can't summon up
the mental energy. In fact, we can barely imagine today
how, during a three-month college vacation, we once
managed to wade through *War and Peace,* Kant's *Cri-
tique of Pure Reason,* and something incomprehensible
by Foucault. And we managed to enjoy it too!

This decline in our willingness to challenge our minds
with difficult new learning goes along with the fact that,
as we age and our short-term memory capacity lessens,
we find such learning more difficult. The combination of
these two factors becomes a vicious circle: on the one
hand, we are less motivated to do the work needed to
exercise our memories by learning new material; on the
other, our failure to develop our brains in this way causes
them to become more resistant to new learning, making
it still harder . . . and, naturally, further demotivating us.
It is truly a fair metaphor to say that our brains rust up.

The problem is that, once our synapses start to become
less conductive, intellectual adventures become harder
and less and less inviting. If we are not careful—and determined—the television will become a drug, the depressant that finally freezes our memories into a single
pattern and more or less assures that we forget everything

outside that restricted sphere that is not fully embedded in our remote memories. Quite as bad, it ensures that we learn little new to expand our horizons.

Of course this situation becomes worse as we age—whether we keep on working, but with less and less challenge and novelty; or whether we retire outright. Perhaps you've spent hours dreaming or planning what you can do when you don't have to spend so many hours, five days a week or more, at the office. Then, again, perhaps you haven't, and retirement sort of crept up on you. Now you don't have anything you have to do. What a relief!

Not really, at least not for many people. For actually the organization and scheduling of our working lives shapes our time, helps us organize, and makes sense of each day, each week, even, by default, each weekend. It motivates us to get certain things done, either because we have to as a condition of our work ("I always have to be at the office by 8:00 A.M."), or because we have to use our nonworking time effectively to get done everything we have to do or would like to do privately ("On Tuesday evening I'll fix the table"; "On Sunday evening I'll watch *Touched by an Angel*").

All those activities give "specialness" to each day, whether or not we realize it. But once you're retired, or for other reasons are unable to do the things you used to do, the activities of one day can be the same as on all the other days. There is little to challenge you. There is little left to remember. Why should you remember them? And so you don't. That means, of course, that you exercise your memory less, and therefore allow more of the electrical circuits in your brain to "silt up." Again, the same vicious downward spiral.

Thus, a third reason for AAMI is a sort of clogging of our electro-synaptic wiring. The solution is to force

ourselves off the television couch and into any more men-
tally challenging endeavor, really anything that provides
a greater mental challenge.

Poor Health, the Wrong Food (and Too Much of It), and the Wrong Nutritional Supplements

There are a number of physical conditions that impair memory performance as well. For example, memory loss can result from such physical disorders as cardiovascular and respiratory problems, diabetes, and a number of neurological disorders. It may also result from drugs and surgical procedures used to treat various medical conditions. We have all heard of an older relative who "was just never the same" after an operation.

Among the drugs that are especially problematic are many substances used to treat sleep disorders, as well as certain antihypertensives and antihistamines. Other physical causes of real or apparent memory loss include chemical imbalances due to malfunctioning glands, and sensory deficiencies (poor sight or hearing).

It is a truism that America is overweight. In fact, some two-thirds of all people over 50 are believed to be ten pounds or more over their ideal weight, and about one-third are bordering on or have crossed over the line into obesity. Couple this with a national nonexercising crisis, and with frequent woeful ignorance of how to eat a nutritionally balanced diet supported by the appropriate augmenting supplements, and it is not surprising that, while we are living longer, we are often doing so with a lot less vitality.

As a result of ever-improving drugs, we are healthier as we age in the sense that we suffer from fewer lethal illnesses (or at least have greatly delayed their onset). But it should not surprise us that our habits of eating poorly, not taking the right nutritional supplements, and not exercising enough tend to make our bodies sluggish, bloated, and somehow more or less permanently feeling slightly queasy. We resort to analgesics and antacids, but we still lack physical energy and enthusiasm. Nor should we be surprised that what de-energizes our bodies does the same thing to our minds and memories. They too feel sluggish and "blah," leaving us slow, undermotivated, and often increasingly depressed. There is simply no doubt that there is a physical-mental connection: as we age, we tend to exercise less and become physically less vital. And that lack of physical vigor saps our mental vigor too—and of course causes our memories to weaken along with the rest.

In addition to the overriding fact that our many poor health habits—from smoking, to excess alcohol consumption, to overeating—harm our memories, there are also specific health and nutritional matters that impact directly on our memory capacity. Of these, the most important (apart from the reduced cellular conductivity discussed above) is lack of sleep. For reasons not fully understood, people who don't get as much sleep as they need show significantly lower cognitive and memory abilities. Of course, lack of sleep affects all activities adversely, but it seems to affect memory considerably more than, say, the ability to carry out tasks requiring fine motor skills, or the capacity for vigorous physical effort.

How much sleep is "enough"? The amount varies with the individual. There is no absolute amount that is a minimum; some people need ten hours a night, others can do fine on half that much. Moreover, the amount of sleep we need tends to decline with age. All you require, then, is enough not to feel tired when you wake up.

Lack of sleep, per se, does not interfere with memory (unless it is caused by sleep apnea, which temporarily cuts off the oxygen supply to your brain, which *does* harm memory). However, tiredness greatly affects our motivation to learn new things, accept new mental challenges, and exercise our memories. It also plays havoc with our ability to concentrate. These reactions greatly harm our memories. Thus, getting enough sleep is most important.

On the positive side, the factors which can help maintain and even help improve our memories include: eating a nutritionally balanced diet; taking the appropriate antioxidants (especially Vitamins A, C, E, and selenium), and boosting the effectiveness of the nutritional phospholipid supplement we recommend by the addition of certain augmenting supplements as we shall discuss in chapter 5.

Thus, a fourth reason for AAMI is generally below-optimum health coupled with insufficient exercise, and insufficient sleep. We can largely overcome these problems by eating correctly, taking the right nutritional supplements, exercising sensibly, and seeing to it we get sufficient sleep.

Stress: Look at It as Fun

Stress tends to interfere with cognitive functioning, and with memory in particular. In addition, stress tends to interfere with sleep, which, as noted, has its own deleterious effect on memory. Therefore, in order to optimize our memory capacity and minimize AAMI, we should eliminate or at least minimize stress.

But the fact is that no one can live without experiencing stress, and many older people, fearful in what seems to be an increasingly aggressive world, tend to be especially stressed. Indeed, by a strange paradox, stress is often a side effect of undertaking those new, unknown, and challenging tasks that help to open our synaptic circuits and keep our memories flowing free. The unknown is generally stressful.

Here, then, is a conundrum: on the one hand, to maintain your memory, you should push into the unknown and seek to conquer possibly dangerous new worlds. On the other hand, doing so will no doubt add stress to your life—particularly if you have not been practicing such efforts for a few years—and stress is bad for your memory.

The solution is not to eliminate stress, but to change your perspective on it. Remember when you used to ski like a wild person, your heart racing at the danger of it? Well, you didn't view that as stress. Rather, the danger was thrilling; you loved the excitement; the adrenaline raced. Probably at those moments all your mental functioning, including your memory, was at a peak.

In the same way, you can—and should—convince yourself that the new mental challenges you are facing as you get older, the new intellectual unknown, is an adventure of the mind. It's fun, every bit as exhilarating as careening down some precipitous, mogul-dotted death slope.

Of course, viewing difficult mental tasks as fun is easier said than done. But it's not at all impossible. Indeed, once you realize that you are causing yourself stress over something that is innately unimportant, such as reading that book the *New York Times* recommended, you will find it much easier to relax about it and perhaps even have a good, healthy laugh at yourself.

Thus, the fifth reason for AAMI is the buildup of stress

*in your life. You can deal with that most effectively—
taking advantage of the clearer perspective age and experience bring—by viewing it not as stress but as a thrill.*

Beat the Blues

At the extreme end of stress, we often find depression.
Of course, that condition interferes with memory, as it
does with most aspects of cognitive and even physical
functioning.

One of the most pervasive problems among the elderly
is depression, from relatively mild to quite severe. Sometimes it is brought on by chemical imbalances in the
brain, but often it is the natural result of the loss of a
loved one, or the loneliness from departed friends. And
little about our physical and mental well-being harms our
ability and willingness to accept new mental challenges—and thus exercise our memories—more than depression.

Severe clinical depression is not something you can
cure or effectively attack yourself. You need prompt and
thorough medical intervention, which is far beyond the
scope of this book. However, a milder form of depression
is sadness, or the "blues." And you can do something
about that.

These are two simple, straightforward steps you can
take to "beat the blues." The first is to force yourself to
do something . . . go out and interact with other people,
wash the car, clean your house. Above all, make a point
of doing something you feel you just don't have the energy to do. You'll be amazed at how quickly your mood
will lift and your energy will return. (And as a bonus,
your house will be clean, too!)

The second approach is to "accentuate the positive,

eliminate the negative." It sounds corny, but if you become aware of your own negative thoughts, and of negative people around you, and learn to avoid both, you will find yourself a great deal happier. Instead, concentrate on thinking about your accomplishments in life, your good friends, the best meal you've ever had. And when your mind tries to drift back to your problems and failures, especially late at night while you're lying awake and your demons want to visit, hold them at bay by reading a cheerful book or remembering your grandchildren at play.

The well-known "Pollyanna tendency" (named for the irrepressibly optimistic heroine in Eleanor Porter's novel *Pollyanna*) holds that we remember pleasant material better than we remember unpleasant material.[37] Exciting, interesting information is stored more easily than that which is dull, partly because we are more alert or pay attention to it more. And our recall of a particular event tends to be better when our present mood matches the mood we were in when the event occurred.

Elizabeth had a terrible fight with Maxine, her best friend of 10 years, and they severed their relationship. Elizabeth was depressed about it for a while but, as time passed and she recovered, she found she couldn't remember many of the details of what happened that day other than that it was "terrible." Several months later Elizabeth's dog was hit by a car and killed. While mourning her dog, Elizabeth once again remembered the events of the day she and Maxine had their fight. The one tragedy had brought to mind the other. This is exactly what depressed people—or, to a lesser extent, people in a blue mood—tend to do. By concentrating on the bad things that are happening, they limit their memories to only previous "bad things." Many studies have shown that self-ratings of memory disturbance by people in a depressed mood are lower than actual performance on memory tests.[38] Of course, this has a further depressing effect. The problem with this sort of selective memory of only the bad is that, since much of life is good, or at worst neutral, people who remember only the bad have a greatly restricted bank of memories on which to call.

Conversely, cheerfully nondepressed people tend to remember a far wider range of events simply because fewer of their memories are blocked off.[39]

Thus, a sixth reason for AAMI is depression and its junior partner, "the blues." The solution—as long as the problem is not too severe—is to challenge yourself with activity, and decide to banish negative thoughts.

These, then, are the six most important inhibitors or destroyers of memory. Fortunately, they can each be attacked and largely resolved, as we shall see in greater detail as we proceed.

I.Q. and Education Make a Difference

One way, on which we have not touched, to slow down memory loss is to be born with a high I.Q. However, in the unlikely event that you have not been able to arrange such a fortunate lineage, you can achieve almost the same protective effect—especially if you are over 75 years old—by having or gaining a high level of education. People with above average education, whether formally acquired at college or during a lifetime of independent study, show relative stability over time on language and other linguistic memory tasks. (On visual-spatial tasks of memory, they showed as much deterioration as persons with low education,[40] probably because these sorts of inputs are less affected by typical education than are verbal skills.) A study conducted at UCLA compared the baseline scores of 42 persons with memory complaints at a three-year follow-up. Level of education and baseline verbal memory were good predictors of change in verbal memory.[41] A study that Dr. Crook participated in with colleagues at the University of Florida showed that on a laboratory test of prose memory, vocabulary mediated the effects of age.[42]

However, if you do not have a high level of education, fret not. Formal education is not the whole story. Researchers at the Mayo Clinic found that, among a group of 161 cognitively normal individuals aged 61 to 100, learning was not only related to level of education.[43] Indeed, many groups of researchers have shown that leading a mentally active life (traveling, reading books, taking courses, pursuing hobbies and new experiences, doing puzzles, expanding your vocabulary, even memorizing the sports scores every day) moderates the unfavorable effects on cognition associated with low education.[44]

❖ MEMORY MOMENT _____

A*ccording to Dr. Alan Baddeley, British psychologist and memory expert, the probability of forgetting something depends on the number of times it is rehearsed or called to mind. The chances of forgetting something only called to mind once are very high.*[45]

3

❖

PS: New Hope for Enhancing Memory

◆

The multitalented PS

◆

If it's natural, why do I need a supplement?

◆

PS charges up cell membranes

◆

Alzheimer's disease (AD) versus age-associated memory impairment (AAMI)

◆

The PS studies summarized

◆

The advantages of soy-based PS

◆

PS is safe

❖

For centuries adventurers and explorers have sought an elusive and magical "fountain of youth." Enticing stories have been written and movies made about their true and fictional efforts. In our heart of hearts, the wistful side of most of us has hoped that such a fountain actually existed, while the more reality-oriented adult side of us knew, with chagrin, that it was not so.

Still, there were individual instances that gave us hope, that showed that aging did not have to be a senility sentence. At a time when the average life expectancy of Greek citizens was 18 years, Pericles, then 69, delivered his Funeral Oration, the foundation of modern democratic thought. Michelangelo began work on the *Pietà Rondanini* when he was almost 80 years old, and Goethe was 84 when Part II of *Faust* was first published.[46]

This chapter documents the true story of what Professor Linus Pauling called an "orthomolecule": a molecule that is "orthodox" to the body, enters it with our normal diet, is familiar with the body's defenses, is seen by them as being of no threat, and is free of all harmful side effects. In fact it is a lipid substance, a unique bio-molecule that can be dissolved both in water and in fats and oils, already found in every cell in the body, but predominantly in brain cells, that is a fail-safe way to turn back the clock for an aging brain. It is the nutritional supplement we have hinted at several times in the last two chapters. It goes by the unwieldy name of *phosphatidylserine* (fos-fa-tid-ill-sereen). Certainly all those adventurers would never have imagined such an unlikely name for their discovery. We call it PS for short.

Available in Europe for years, phosphatidylserine, PS, "bathes" and rejuvenates the membranes of brain cells. Dr. Parris M. Kidd, an internationally recognized cell biologist and authority on nutrition and human health, who works closely with Lucas Meyer, the manufacturer of almost the entire world's supply of PS, and many other nutritional supplement components, calls it the "single best means for conserving memory and other higher brain functions."[47] And Dr. Crook, whose international research team has conducted comprehensive research in literally dozens of leading universities on virtually every drug developed during the past twenty years to treat AAMI, has joined Brenda Adderly in writing this book because, as he states flatly, "PS is by far the best of all the drugs and nutritional supplements we have ever tested for retarding Age-Associated Memory Impairment (AAMI)."

The use of PS is, of course, the centerpiece of *The Memory Cure,* our own adventure in seeking that rare elixir to turn back the ravages of time. And, just as Dorothy and her friends in the land of Oz found that what they were each seeking was within themselves all the time, so it is true for PS.

The Multitalented PS

Within our bodies, PS is most heavily concentrated in the internal layer of the membranes of brain cells. Not only does the membrane act as a structural support, defining the extension of the cell in all its directions; but, more importantly, it is directly and actively involved in conducting information across the synaptic gap from one cell to another.

PS acts on multiple neurochemical systems. It increases the action of receptors located on the target cell's membranal surface, and it stimulates the production and release of specific neurotransmitters, namely epinephrine, norepinephrine, serotonin, and dopamine. Several studies have hinted that PS activates dopamine[48] and serotonin[49] pathways in nonsenile humans, as well as in patients affected with presenile dementia. In other words,

PS is essential for influencing the neurotransmitters that help pass messages from one cell to another and, therefore, for a good memory.

By restoring the activity of PS in aging cell membranes with a PS supplement, we keep the chemical interaction and the transfer of electrical impulses between neurons more open at both the sending and receiving ends. Thus, *new* information can more easily carve a new pattern of electrical transmission in our brains, and be more easily converted into *remembered* information. Our memories are reinvigorated—perhaps to be "as good as new."

If It's Natural, Why Do I Need a Supplement?

Small amounts of PS do exist in common foods like fish, rice, soy products, and green leafy vegetables, and PS is an essential part of our diet. The problem is that it's difficult to get enough PS through our food to jump-start the aging cells in our brain. As with so many aspects of aging, since we were not evolutionarily programmed to live into old age, the amounts of PS we take in from our normal food intake, while sufficient to serve our needs up to early middle age (a full lifetime in prehistoric times) are not sufficient to satisfy our needs in later life. That's why we need supplemental PS which, happily, acts just like the PS we eat in our food.

Taken orally, PS is rapidly absorbed and readily crosses the blood-brain barrier, a natural biochemical protector that surrounds all the capillaries in the brain and prevents harmful substances from "leaking out" of the bloodstream into the brain. When mice were intravenously injected with radioisotopic PS (to distinguish it from that made by the body), it was absorbed into the brain tissues within minutes. Evaluation of separate brain areas showed that most substantial quantities of PS were present in the cortex, hippocampus, and hypothalamus, thus ensuring that the areas known to be centrally involved with memory were being adequately supplied with the supplement.[50]

PS is important to individual cells in a number of ways:

◆ The outermost layer of the cell, the membrane— which is particularly high in PS—helps control the entry of nutrients into the cell and the exit of waste products. Proteins in the membrane, which rely on PS to maintain their full functional capacity, transform the membrane into a kind of master switch for the cell to help in cell movement, and shape changes such as flattening or expansion of the cell.

◆ In addition to the cell-to-cell communication mentioned above, proteins also assist the cell in sending along chemical or electrical "messages" from the outside of the cell to its interior.

To date, over sixty human studies of PS have been published in peer-review journals, of which almost a third were placebo-controlled, double-blind (the gold standard of academic research). They consistently show that PS can turn back the clock in the nondiseased aging brain and revitalize its memory functions. In addition:

◆ PS can help the individual cope with stress.

◆ PS helps normalize brain biochemistry and physiology at every level.

◆ PS is safe to take and has no reported adverse effects.

As Dr. Kidd writes, "With almost 3,000 peer-reviewed research papers available on PS, science has some understanding of how it works. It is the single best nutrient (really, the single best means of any kind) for safely conserving and restoring crucial higher functions of the brain (what is considered cognition). The remarkable benefits of PS and its safety in use are now established beyond doubt. What remains is to spread the message to the people who can benefit from PS."[51]

PS Charges Up Cell Membranes

As we age, the composition of the membranes of our brain cells changes in several ways. One of the important changes is that the membranes become loaded with cholesterol, making some brain cells less fluid.[52] It is likely that the rigid membranes of these cholesterol-laden cells are less receptive to impulses from other neurons. And that interferes with the retrieval of memories.

Just as our bodies require food to regain energy when we are weary, the membranes of our aging nerve cells need a boost to help them regain their natural activity, and it is likely that PS provides this boost.[53] The cell membranes are revitalized and allow nutrients to enter the cell more easily, as they did when they were "younger."

You don't have to take our word for it that PS can halt the decline in memory. In the balance of this chapter we'll take a look at some of the many studies that have been done on PS, both in this country and abroad, to prove that PS is a crucial element in halting or reversing AAMI.

A phosphorus-containing lipid substance, i.e., a phospholipid, PS was first chemically isolated by J. Folch in 1948.[54] After European researchers found a way to extract and concentrate PS from the brains of cattle, they began conducting research, mainly centering around its effect in the brain.

Early studies examining the effects of PS were done with rats that had sustained cerebral damage. For instance, to find out whether PS derived from the extracted and purified bovine brain cortex could prevent age-dependent cerebral dysfunctions, researchers in Italy added it to the drinking water of a group of aging rats. Nineteen months later, the rats were tested for their ability to learn how to avoid an electric shock in a "shuttle" box. PS definitely prevented a decline in the learning capability of the aged rats. Examination of their brains at 27 months showed that PS prevented certain specific age-induced changes in the hippocampus.[55]

In an interview for a British newspaper, Dr. Kidd aptly summarized 11 years of animal research by saying, "As laboratory rats reach middle age, they are less able to negotiate mazes [indicating a loss of spatial memory]. If they take PS, they stay smart into old age."[56] One Italian researcher reported the results of his studies as showing that PS "completely prevents" the decline of learning capability that occurs in aged rats.[57]

During the early 1980s, a great deal of exploratory research on the effects of PS on humans was conducted, mostly in Italy. These studies involved only small numbers of people, and were not intended to provide rigorous, double-blind, placebo-controlled proof. Rather they were used, as early research often is, to give investigators ideas about where more sophisticated research should best be aimed.

No one knows to what degree these factors bias or change the results of a study, but because they might exert influence, studies that don't control for them are obviously not as valuable as double-blind, placebo-con-

trolled studies where neither patients nor doctors know
who is receiving the drug under study. Nevertheless, such
exploratory trials are extremely valuable as a first step in
determining the effects of a new medication or supplement, in encouraging later researchers to put the time and
money into designing more rigorous research, and in giving clues as to what to look for.

Given that caveat, it's worth examining some of the
promising results that the Italian researchers discovered,
each of which contributed to the growing information
about the effects of PS. Unless otherwise noted, participants were treated with 300 milligrams of PS daily, administered in three 100-milligram doses with meals.

◆ **Attention, Memory, and Mood Improve with
PS.** In 1987, researchers selected 30 individuals (21 men,
9 women with an average age of 69 years) with mild
cognitive and behavioral deterioration from either hospital or outpatient groups. After being given an extensive
series of attention/concentration and memory tests, and
being rated on behavioral scales, participants received
300 milligrams of PS daily for two months, after which
they were retested. For one attention/concentration test
involving crossing out randomly interspersed target letters C and E on a sheet of paper, they were rated significantly higher. In the memory tests, acquisition of new
memory, recall of verbal memory, and immediate semantic memory were significantly improved, as was mood.[58]

◆ **PS Significantly Improves Memory,** especially in
those with a moderate degree of impairment. From a private nursing home in Rome in 1987, 35 patients (19
males, 16 females) ranging in age from 61 to 80 years,
were treated with 300 milligrams of PS daily for two
months. Patients showing advanced stages of dementia
or presenting medical or psychiatric diseases were ex-

cluded. The group was tested on a series of memory tests and a behavioral rating scale three times: at the beginning of the study, at the thirtieth day, and at the end of the PS treatment. All tests showed highly significant improvement, but the best results were obtained with patients who had only a moderate degree of impairment. The authors noted that PS may make the elderly person more receptive to environmental stimuli, resulting in increased socialization and initiative, which, in turn, results in increased adaptation and participation in daily activities.[59]

◆ **PS Significantly Improves the Ability to Learn Lists of Words,** as well as attentive and visual-perceptive abilities. PS was given orally to 30 men and 4 women (ranging in age from 62 to 76 years). The number of years of schooling ranged from 3 to 8, with an average of 4.6 years. Only nine of the group had normal brain scans, while 24 showed a mild reduction in the size of the cortex, and 19 showed a slight enlargement of cerebral ventricles. Patients were tested four different times: at the beginning of the study, after 30 days, after 60 days, and 30 days after the end of the daily treatment regimen of 300 milligrams of PS. A significant improvement occurred in the learning of lists of 15 words and in being able to remember, and in a digit symbol test that measured attentive and visual-perceptive abilities. When treatment was ended, most test scores tended back toward the baseline levels obtained before treatment.[60]

◆ **PS Has a Lasting Effect on Cognitive and Behavioral Functions.** When 27 Italian outpatients with mild "senile cognitive decline" were treated with 300 milligrams of PS for 60 days, there was improvement in cognitive and behavioral functions (self-sufficiency, better sleep, initiative, and socialization). The interesting thing about this study, however, is that the improvement continued for a month after the end of therapy.[61]

Alzheimer's Disease (AD) versus Age-Associated Memory Impairment (AAMI)

Before we proceed to discuss all of the human research that supports the efficacy of PS, we should touch briefly on the frightening subject of Alzheimer's disease (AD). As we have described earlier, while AD is a horrifying disease, it does not strike a high percentage of the population until quite late in life. Nevertheless, ignoring percentages, it does attack and debilitate a frighteningly large number of people. Therefore, it is not unreasonable for everyone who shows early signs of a declining memory to worry whether they are, in fact, showing the early signs of AD.

From that worrying thought, we move on to the next one, namely whether all memory loss is actually the start of a long continuum down the slide to eventual AD. In other words, will we all get the disease if we live long enough (even if "long enough" means reaching some unattainable age); and is the difference between those who do and those who don't exhibit the full symptoms of AD before they die at a normally attainable age merely a difference in the speed of AD's advance? Or, alternatively, are AAMI and AD on a different continuum, the former a symptom of ordinary aging, the latter a true disease?

Opinions on this score vary widely. For our part, we tend to believe that there is at least some degree of continuum between the two and that the line between AAMI in its more severe manifestations and AD in its milder forms is a largely arbitrary one. As Caroline McNeil, Public Information Officer of the National Institutes of

Health, wrote in a 1991 National Institute on Aging booklet, "We know that Alzheimer's begins in the entorhinal cortex and proceeds to the *hippocampus,* a way station important in memory formation. It then gradually spreads to other regions, particularly the *cerebral cortex.* This is the outer area of the brain, which is involved in functions such as language and reason. In the regions attacked by Alzheimer's, the nerve cells or *neurons* degenerate, losing their connections or *synapses* with other neurons. Some neurons die."[62] You will immediately note that this description sounds very much the same, albeit more extreme, as the one that would apply to "ordinary" memory loss.

AD can only be definitively diagnosed posthumously when an autopsy finds twisted strands of fiber inside the brain and widespread deposits of amyloid plaques. (For living patients AD can only be diagnosed symptomatically.) These neurofibrillary tangles and amyloid plaques are the most fundamental symptoms of full-blown AD. However, to a lesser degree, these tangles and plaques are found in the brains of very old people who have not been diagnosed with AD.

If you accept our view that AD is the extreme case of normal AAMI, then it follows that, by halting, delaying, and/or mitigating the onset of AAMI, PS may also delay the onset of AD in those relatively few individuals who will go on to develop the disorder.

However, we would not go so far as to claim or even suggest that PS cures AD. (And neither has Dr. Kidd.) Even if PS helps a little, by the time a patient's mind has degenerated enough to be diagnosed with AD, the degree of improvement one might expect from PS will fall far short of the improvement that would be needed to achieve anything close to a cure.

We should point out, moreover, that our feeling that AD is essentially an exaggeration of AAMI is not shared by many respected experts in the field and remains a controversial and largely unproven view. Nevertheless, in reviewing all the copious research on PS, we have included the key studies both on AD patients and on subjects whose memory impairment falls well short of the AD level. It is not surprising to us that positive effects of PS were also seen in AD, although the effects were generally less profound than in AAMI. After all, in heart disease, cancer, and most other medical disorders, the importance of early detection and treatment is fully appreciated. If, as we believe, AAMI and AD lie on a continuum in terms of clinical symptoms, both structural brain changes and chemical changes in the brain, then waiting to make a diagnosis of AD before starting treatment on AAMI is like waiting for a heart attack before starting treatment of coronary heart disease.

The thesis of this book is that PS can slow, halt, or reverse the decline of memory due to normal aging. The following double-blind, placebo-controlled research, considered as a whole body of work, amply proves that this thesis is correct. No other product ever researched has shown similar effectiveness.

The PS Studies Summarized

Here, then, is a partial list of the studies on PS. We judge each to be methodologically sound and therefore persuasive in its own right. Taken together, we believe the results of these studies are compelling. Since they lie at the heart of the Memory Cure we are recommending in this book, we will cover them in some detail.

◆ **PS Is Effective in Improving a Range of Cogni-**

tive Abilities. The first carefully controlled, double-blind study conducted on PS was by P. J. Delwaide and three co-researchers at the respected University of Liège in Belgium. Published in 1986, this study examined 35 people, aged 65 to 91, hospitalized with mild to moderate memory impairment due to AD. The patients were given memory tests at the start of the trial and then took 300 milligrams of PS for six weeks. They were evaluated at the start of the study, after three and six weeks, and a fourth time three weeks after the end of the study.

The patients were tested across a broad range of cognitive abilities covering everything from communication skills to bowel control. When these various evaluations were condensed into ten groupings, small but meaningful improvements were observed in all ten categories. Clearly, this study predicted the results of the many later ones, namely that, while PS cannot cure AD, it is useful even in that sad and extreme condition.

◆ **PS Repeats Earlier Improvements in Cognitive Function.** In 1987, Professor Villardita, of the University of Catania in Italy, conducted a sophisticated, randomized, double-blind, placebo-controlled study of 170 patients who had moderate cognitive deterioration. Half the patients were given 300 milligrams of PS daily for 90 days; the other half received a placebo. The participants were between the ages of 55 to 80 years (average age of 65) and were patients in three different Italian medical centers. To assess changes in cognitive function, patients were evaluated with neuropsychological tests at the beginning of the study, after 45 days, and again after 90 days. A wide range of tests was administered to these patients, covering both memory and various types of cognitive function. In almost every test, the PS patients clearly outscored the controls. On memory, the results were especially impressive: out of five tests conducted, each showed a substantial improvement, with the improvement among the PS patients continuing relative to the placebo group throughout the 90-day period. Of special importance was the fact that patients treated with PS showed a significant improvement in semantic association ability and in verbal fluency.[63] The chart below makes the degree of improvement clear.

◆ **PS Greatly Improves Attention and Concentration** in patients with AD. In a separate study conducted in the same year by G. Palmieri, R. Palmieri, et al., also in Italy, patients with AD were studied in three clinical centers in different Italian cities (Milan, Brescia, and Padua), with separate randomization for each center. The 87 patients (30 males, 57 females) were, on the average, 73 years old. Forty-three were in the placebo group and 44 in the active drug group. The patients were assessed with neuropsychological, behavioral, and memory tests conducted at the beginning of the study, at the end of the

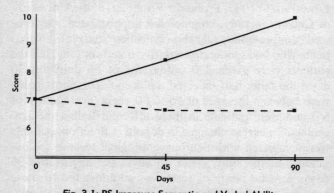

Fig. 3.1: PS Improves Semantic and Verbal Ability
Over a three-month period, patients were treated with PS (solid line) or a placebo (dotted line). At three different dates, their memory was tested.

60-day treatment period, and again 30 days after treatment was discontinued. The results of a five-word memory test were particularly impressive. There could be no doubt that the PS had greatly improved things. Beyond that, however, it was also clear that self-sufficiency, orientation, apathy, and withdrawal all improved significantly for the group taking PS, as did scores on attention and concentration. All of these, of course, contribute to improved memory.[64]

◆ **PS Is Beneficial with Early-stage Alzheimer's Patients.** The Palmieris' study was duplicated in 1987 by another group of Italian investigators led by D. Nerozzi. Again, this was double-blind, placebo-controlled research. It involved 35 patients diagnosed with early-stage AD, 60 to 80 years old, recruited from retirement homes around Rome.

The patients received 300 milligrams of PS daily for 60 days. The results, as with the Palmieris' study, showed a statistically significant benefit on delayed memory recollection.[65]

◆ **PS Significantly Helps Patients with Alzheimer's Disease.** In 1988 a group of 22 Italian researchers led by L. Amaducci from seven different neurological research centers throughout Italy conducted a double-blind, randomized, placebo-controlled study involving 142 patients. Collectively their continuing studies are known as the Italian Multicenter Study of Dementia (Studio Multicentrico Italiano sulla Demenza). Their work in this particular study attempted to replicate the positive PS findings of the other studies described earlier with respect to AD.

For three months the patients, aged 40 to 80 (average age 62), received either 200 milligrams daily (in 100-milligram capsules taken at meals) of PS or a placebo, with a follow-up period of 21 months (a total of 24 months). Paitents were evaluated prior to treatment, at the end of the three-month treatment period, and at six-month intervals thereafter until the 24 months was reached. Results at the three- and six-month follow-up periods showed that differences between the PS and placebo groups were significant. Scores on personal memory, overall memory, and performance of everyday activities were significantly improved. Those with severe impairment who took the placebo deteriorated significantly during the first six months, while those treated with PS improved during the same period.[66]

◆ **PS Improves Memory Skills in Patients with AAMI.** A 1991 study conducted by a group of American researchers led by Dr. Crook compared the effects of phosphatidylserine to a placebo on 149 persons, ages 50 to 75, who demonstrated typical symptoms of AAMI, but not AD. Colleagues at Vanderbilt University School of Medicine in Nashville, Tennessee, and at Stanford University in Palo Alto, California, along with those at Dr. Crook's Memory Assessment Clinic in Bethesda, Maryland, took great care to exclude persons with symptoms of medical disorders, depression, stroke, or other brain damage, in the double-blind, randomized, placebo-controlled comparison.

Study participants took either 300 milligrams of PS (100 milligrams three times daily) or an inert placebo for 12 weeks. A sophisticated neuropsychological test battery was administered at 3, 6, 9, and 12 weeks and performance was compared to that at the beginning of the study. Those who took PS demonstrated a 30 percent improvement in cognitive function, including memory, learning, and recalling names, faces, and numbers.

An important finding from this trial was that an analysis of subgroups suggested that persons within the sample who performed at a relatively low level prior to treatment were most likely to respond to PS. Within this subgroup, there also was specific improvement on such memory components as recognizing faces, learning and remembering names and faces, remembering telephone numbers and a paragraph recently read, and concentrating while reading, conversing, or performing tasks.

The data on the subtest that measured the ability to remember the name of someone to whom one is introduced proved so significant that Dr. Crook and his colleagues considered it a "model" to consider the positive effects of PS. By looking at the expected decline on the test from the normative data on several thousand subjects, they were able to conclude that PS had prevented the equivalent of 12 years of memory decline.[67]

◆ **PS Improves Symptoms in Patients with AD.** In 1992, Dr. Crook and colleagues at Vanderbilt University published their study of 51 patients between the ages of 55 and 85 years who met the clinical criteria for AD. In a double-blind, randomized, placebo-controlled comparison that lasted for 12 weeks, patients received either 300 milligrams (100 milligrams three times daily) of PS or a placebo. Patients were evaluated at the beginning of the study and at three-week intervals during the study. The results showed that memory improved although considerably less than seen in the AAMI study, with the improvement clearest in patients in the early stages of AD. Clearly, no one will conclude that PS is a cure for AD. In general, the results showed that PS exerts a mild and subtle therapeutic effect in AD for those who have not progressed to the middle and later stages of the disorder.[68]

◆ **PS Improves Behavioral and Cognitive Func-**

tions. Yet another impressive study was conducted in 1992 by T. Cenacchi leading a long and impressive list of Italian investigators. In this large study, 494 patients were recruited from 23 geriatric or general medicine hospital units in northern Italy, and were examined just before starting therapy, and three and six months thereafter. The effect of 300 milligrams of PS administered daily was compared to a placebo.

Memory, learning, and other cognitive abilities were measured, as were the effects of PS on routine activities of daily life. The researchers concluded, in typically contained academic language, that "statistically significant improvements in the phosphatidylserine-treated group compared to placebo were observed both in terms of behavioral and cognitive parameters. . . . These results are clinically important since the patients were representative of the geriatric population commonly met in clinical practice."[69]

◆ **PS Improves Scores on Wechsler Intelligence Test.** Finally, a study was completed in 1995 in Israel. Fifty-seven elderly persons (aged 60 to 80 years) living in three kibbutzim (collective communities) were randomly assigned to a treatment or placebo group and received 300 milligrams of plant-derived PS mixed with lecithin, or 500 milligrams of lecithin only as a placebo.

The results of this trial showed that both placebo and treatment groups showed significant improvement in the total score on an intelligence test (Wechsler), but only for the PS group were there significant changes in eight of the nine components of the test. Further, those persons who scored higher to begin with on the memory scale showed significant memory improvements, whereas those who had scored lower did not (possibly because they were already in the early stages of an undiagnosed dementing disease). One of the serendipitous findings of the study—due to the fact that it was begun in late summer and extended into the winter months—was that "winter blues" (depressive symptoms) increased significantly for the placebo group while there was no change in mood for the PS group.[70]

Although there appears to be some doubt about this, we are informed that the PS used in this research was derived from white cabbage, and was neither bovine nor soy derived. As we shall discuss below, the efficacy of soy-derived PS is comparable to or perhaps even greater than that of PS derived from cattle. However, no studies have been conducted to compare these types of PS and PS extracted from cabbage. Thus, it remains possible that the significant but somewhat less impressive results of this study may be due to the use of lower-efficacy PS.

By the early 1990s, the focus of AAMI research on PS and other compounds had shifted to the United States, largely due to the efforts of Dr. Crook and his associates at the Memory Assessment Clinic (MAC) in Bethesda, Maryland, and Scottsdale, Arizona. MAC has working affiliations with more than 50 academic research centers in the United States and 10 European countries. After dozens of large-scale, multi-center, clinical trials, PS proved the most effective compound for the treatment of AAMI.

The Advantages of Soy-Based PS

As questions arose about the safety factors of PS generated from cattle, the lead manufacturer of the product spearheaded a move to generate the supplement from soybeans. This proved feasible. However, to make sure that the product was identical to the earlier bovine PS,

Dr. Crook conducted a comparative study between the two. Looking at four important memory abilities—remembering names immediately after introduction, learning and remembering written information, recognizing someone previously seen, and dialing a 10-digit telephone number from memory—Dr. Crook found that the soy-based PS product (Leci-PS™) is clearly as effective as the bovine product in all respects involving memory. There is even some indication that in reversing age-related memory loss and for some memory skills, the soy product may be more effective. (See charts on pages 87 and 88.)

PS Is Safe

PS has been used for over twenty years in Italy. The supplement is available and widely used throughout the United States, Europe, and many other parts of the world. Millions of people are taking it regularly. Dozens of human studies using PS have been conducted in universities in the United States and worldwide. Dr. Crook himself has conducted research among over 500 patients.

The Cenacchi group also kept track of more than 450 patients, and found that PS did not interact with the pharmaceutical drugs their patients were taking. During that entire experience base, no negative side effects of any sort have been reported.

Summary: PS Works

All this research should leave you in no doubt that phosphatidylserine (PS) is effective in delaying and in usually reversing AAMI. The charts shown here make the point as clearly as any words we could write.

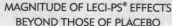

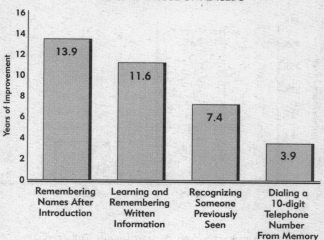

MAGNITUDE OF LECI-PS® EFFECTS
BEYOND THOSE OF PLACEBO

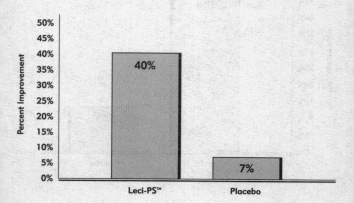

IMPROVEMENT AFTER TWELVE WEEKS TREATMENT
LEARNING AND REMEMBERING WRITTEN INFORMATION

IMPROVEMENT AFTER TWELVE WEEKS TREATMENT
REMEMBERING NAMES ONE HOUR AFTER INTRODUCTION

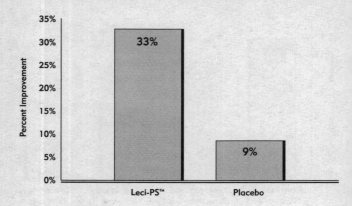

IMPROVEMENT AFTER TWELVE WEEKS TREATMENT
REMEMBERING NAMES IMMEDIATELY AFTER INTRODUCTION

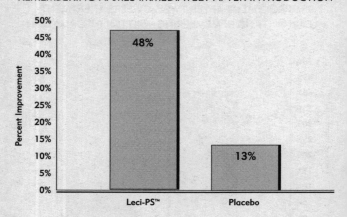

Dr. Paris Kidd, a leading expert in cell biology and nutrition, in connection with his work on behalf of Lucas Meyer, conducted a careful review of all the published research papers that have investigated the effects of PS (only some of which are summarized above) and reported: "It is not a scientific exaggeration to conclude from the extensive research on PS, that it benefits virtually every brain function that can be tested."[71] We fully agree with Dr. Kidd that PS slows, halts, or reverses AAMI.

As a final note, buyer beware: phosphorylated serine—also available as a dietary supplement—does not work like PS. It is not a phospholipid, and consumers report it can cause highly uncomfortable adverse reactions.[72] So be sure you get the real thing. It works!

4

❖❖

The Six-Step Memory Cure

Step 1: Take a PS supplement

◆

Step 2: Exercise your mind

◆

*Step 3: Protect your health, eat a healthy diet,
add PS-boosting supplements*

◆

Step 4: Change your attitude toward stress

◆

Step 5: Exercise to maintain your overall health

◆

Step 6: Maintain a positive attitude

❖❖

The replacement of PS in supplement form is the most crucial step in halting and reversing age-related memory decline. If you did nothing else, you would almost certainly improve your memory or at least halt its decline. However, to obtain the supplement's full effectiveness, it should be incorporated into a more complete memory-enhancement program. For while just taking a

PS pill daily will help alleviate memory loss, taking PS in conjunction with a full memory enhancement program will lead to truly dramatic results for most people. Our simple, six-step plan is designed to maximize your memory and minimize or eliminate any symptoms of AAMI from which you have suffered or may be anticipating.

THE 6-STEP MEMORY CURE PROGRAM

1   Take a PS supplement daily in the recommended dosage.

2   Exercise your mind to enhance your memory skills, and learn more to enlarge your bank of knowledge from which to draw memories.

3   Protect your health, eat a healthy diet, add PS-boosting supplements.

4   Change your attitude toward stress.

5   Maintain your overall health, and exercise regularly.

6   Maintain a positive attitude.

Popular writers on memory tend to talk about it as if it were like a muscle—the more you exercise it the stronger (or bigger) it gets. Up to a point, there is some validity to this idea. Certainly, exercising our memories opens up the conductivity of the channels in our brains, which defines them. However, we must take care to remember that memory is not a simple, isolated entity that can be exercised independently, comparable to, say, your biceps, which get bigger and stronger as you work them. Rather, memory is a compilation of many processes, each of which is affected by different factors in the way the body functions. In order to offset AAMI, we therefore have to attend to more than just practicing our memorization skills, important though that is. Let's take a closer look at each of the six steps that make up our Memory Cure program.

STEP 1

Take a PS Supplement

Obviously, PS is the heart of the Memory Cure. Taken orally, it is absorbed rapidly and readily crosses the blood-brain barrier to reach the brain, where it begins to act on the cell membranes. Dosages depend on your condition, but generally we recommend that you begin with 200–300 milligrams daily for 30 days, taking a dose of 100 milligrams twice or three times a day. This should provide enough PS to saturate your cell membranes initially. Thereafter, you can probably switch to a daily 100 milligram maintenance level. One hundred milligrams is sufficient for people in their forties and fifties who have not yet experienced much memory loss and intend to take PS prophylactically. Older people who already have significant AAMI may wish to continue at the 300 milligrams per day dosage level. There is no evidence that, even at double this level (which we do not recommend), there are any side effects. And studies with laboratory animals show no toxicity at dosage levels that represent the equivalent of several times the 300 mg per day human dose level.[73] Thus, apart from the extra cost of taking the larger quantity, there are no disadvantages to doing so. For most people, it takes about 21 days for any improvement to start to become noticeable, and the improvement can be expected to continue for several months before leveling. In order to maintain the benefits of PS, you will have to continue taking it indefinitely, much as you have to have an adequate nutritional intake every day.

There is no evidence that PS is inappropriate for pregnant women. However, given that no research has been done in this area and that, in any case, they are likely to be too young to be experiencing significant AAMI, we recommend against the use of PS during pregnancy or lactation. We also suggest that, if you are taking anticoagulant medications, you advise your doctor *before* taking PS.

You can purchase PS at almost any health-food store or in the health-food section of almost any drugstore. A few supermarkets also carry PS.

The supplement is available in two forms. The most common is a pill or gel capsule. There are over 100 different products on the market, produced by many different manufacturers.

To be sure the pills contain the right type and quantity of PS, however, we recommend that you purchase: either a product manufactured by Sundown, Thompson or Rexall, which are all part of the same large, reliable nutritional supplements company; or any product that carries the Leci-PS™ logo, which means that the products' raw material content has been checked by Lucas Meyer, which manufactures most of the PS sold and is also a large and reliable firm. (Note: You may have trouble finding their logo on bottles since it is often quite small and difficult to read.)

STEP 2

Exercise Your Mind to Enhance Your
Memory Skills

As our brains become "set in their ways," we tend to work less hard at remembering. If the channel is clogged, why try to navigate it? Our Memory Cure program enhances the effect of PS supplements through "channel-opening" exercises.

Good memory is partly an acquired skill, as attested to by the experience of working actors. Many of them can learn vast, complicated parts with remarkable speed. However, since few of the rest of us have ever had that sort of perfect memory, most of us can benefit from the Memory Maximizer strategies contained in chapter 5. Even for those of us who are satisfied with our memories, it is worthwhile to consider a few fairly simple and quick techniques that can give our memories a considerable boost.

Of course, mice are mice and (notwithstanding the clichéd question, "Are you a man or a mouse?") humans are humans. It is instructive, therefore, to wonder whether the same phenomenon can be seen among us.

An interesting example showing precisely this phenomenon at work was a series of tests, administered by Dr. Crook's staff, to which Hugh Downs, the cohost of *20/20*, submitted himself on prime-time television. While Downs is, of course, well known to everyone, it may surprise you that he has had more network television exposure than any other person to date. Thus, over the years, he has obviously been remarkably well trained in dealing with a mass of confusing input, coming from his control room via his earpiece, his guests, his own notes, the Tele-PrompTer, cue cards, and his observation of surrounding—often frenetic—events.

When Downs was tested for memory and various forms of cognitive ability, the results showed that, relative to even young adults, he was above average on virtually all scores, and in one case, where the test involved memorizing verbal information while dealing with multiple distractions, he obtained the highest score ever recorded—even among thousands of 18- to 21-year-old college students!

Autopsies on healthy people who died from causes other than brain problems show that the neurons' dendritic branches keep growing and continue to make new connections even in old age.[74] A 1997 study conducted at the Salk Institute for Biological Studies by Drs. Fred H. Gage, Gerd Kempermann, and H. George Kuhn shows that brain enrichment increased learning in laboratory mice. While a number of previous studies, notably the pioneering work of neuroanatomist Dr. Marian Diamond, have shown the same effect, the biological reasons behind it have been hotly debated. In the Salk study, mice were separated into two groups. One group was housed in a standard-sized cage containing food and water. The other group was housed in a large cage with the same food and water supply, but "enriched" with tunnels, toys, and an exercise wheel. After 40 days, the two groups were compared in a water maze test and, as expected from previously published studies, the mice in the enriched environment performed significantly better.

When they examined the brains of the animals, the researchers found that the hippocampi of the "enriched" mice contained an average of 40,000 more nerve cells than those of the control group. Since brain cells seem to have divided at the same rate in both groups, the researchers don't think the enhanced performance occurred because the mice in the enriched group generated more brain cells. Instead, a cerebrally enriched environment appears to foster the *survival* of new brain cells.

Several days before the experiment's end, some of the mice were injected with a dye that would make new brain cells fluorescent so that they could be seen under a microscope. In the enriched animals, the survival rate of newborn cells was 60 percent higher than in the control group. The authors think the results are particularly remarkable because the experiments were not carried out in infant mice, but in adult animals. Dr. Gage, the senior author, thinks this shows that intellectual stimulation during life's later years can still influence the "architecture" of the brain.[75] In other words, he underlines our conviction that, at any age, the *ability* to remember can be improved.

Enriching your own environment might mean taking a class, participating in a discussion group on current events, or joining a book club. If groups aren't "your thing," then reading a serious magazine or a challenging book will help exercise your mind, although you'll find it more stimulating if you can discuss what you've read with someone else.

Other activities that keep us mentally alert include playing games that tap into memory, such as bridge, chess, or Trivial Pursuit. If you don't like games, even television quiz shows can test your memory or help you to learn new facts. (But remember to turn off your television after the quiz show is over!) Learn to use a computer; this is a challenge at any age. Think you're too old? The mother of one acquaintance bought her first computer at the age of 81, and she now uses it every day to play games and find new recipes on the Internet. She even bought a computer program to help her learn Spanish. She's living proof that the old adage "you can't teach an old dog new tricks" is just plain wrong.

Actually, it doesn't matter what new material you choose to learn. Memorizing statistics from the sports page, or following your team's progress in its league each day, can have a clear positive effect on your memory. You don't have to be a chess grand master to benefit from exercising your mind. All that does matter is that what you decide to work at mentally is something that is relevant to you so that you are motivated to keep at it . . . and that you *do* keep at it. Exercising your mind is an important way of enhancing the effectiveness of PS.

MAKE A COMMITMENT TO IMPROVE MEMORY SKILLS

An important component of forgetting or of poor memory skills may be that you never felt it emotionally important that you make a commitment to change. Yes, it's aggravating when you can't find your eyeglasses or the current issue of *TV Guide,* but we've heard too many people say, "I don't know what I did with it" and/or "I guess I'm just getting old and forgetful." In our experience of working with people who think they have a poor memory, we rarely hear them say, "I'm going to fix this situation. I'm going to learn what I need to do and *do* it."

 MEMORY MOMENT _____

> " It takes more than a good memory to have a good memory."
>
> —Anonymous.

It takes time to develop a better memory. You can't become really skilled at it quickly any more than you can become a star athlete or a skilled painter overnight. So, the first step is to decide, and really mean it, that you are going to fix the situation. The next step is to start to pay attention to how it is you lose things or what it is you do—or more likely, don't do—that enables you to forget important things. This observational task in itself will probably reduce forgetting to some extent. But that's not all you want. You want to reorganize and prevent it from repeating.

Answering the following questions will help you begin to think about your "forgetful behavior" and, importantly, will allow you to measure objectively how forgetful you really are. By repeating the process every few months, you can keep track of how you are progressing in improving your memory. You should, of course, tailor your self-questionnaire to your own behavior patterns. However, here are some examples from a typical list of the questions you might develop for yourself:

1 (If you are a gardener, collector, bird-watcher, or the like.) How many of the Latin names of the plants in my garden, or the technical descriptions of the items in my collection, can I remember as I look at them? You can give yourself a time limit, say 15 minutes, so that the test is comparable each time you do it.

2 How many news-article subjects can you remember from this morning's paper? This test should be conducted at the same time each afternoon or evening.

3 (If you are a businessperson.) Make out a list of, say, ten key business numbers (e.g., certain stock market quotes, the Dow Jones and other stock mar-

ket averages) and see how many of those you can
recall. Again, give yourself the test at about the
same time of the day.
4 Of all the people you've talked to in the last, say,
seven days, how many can you recall by name?

You can make this test as long or as short as you like,
but do write down the items in your test so that you can
test your abilities against the same challenges each time
you repeat the trial. As you strive to repeat it, say, once
every three months, you will almost certainly see an improvement in your performance. This will mean two
things: you are exercising your mind more and getting
better at using it to remember; and the PS you are taking
is kicking in. Some experts will tell you that a good part
of the improvement stems from your being aware that
you are doing something to create an improvement in
your memory. Possibly. But ignore them! It's an improvement, isn't it? What more do you want?

HELP YOUR MEMORY OUT

Before we leave the subject of improving your memory by exercising your mind, let us add the thought that
you can also augment the *effectiveness* of your memory
by adopting certain techniques for compensating for any
memory declines you may not have been able to avoid:

◆ Take notes. This is obvious; if you write it down,
you won't forget it. However, one friend has improved his note-taking need from being a necessary but annoying chore to a valuable business aid.
Instead of taking notes for himself, he confirms everything he wants to remember in a letter. Of
course, those letters help him to remember. "But
what is much more useful," he explains with a

rather sly grin, "is that my letters make sure the other fellow can't forget either!"

◆ Write down things you want to remember right away. An author friend has discovered that, no matter how good an idea she has, if she doesn't write it down right then, she won't remember it the next day when she sits down at her computer. She has little notebooks with pages that tear out easily situated at all the places where she is most likely to have an idea: next to the bed, next to the couch where she reads and watches television, and on a small table next to the bathtub because she has discovered that while she is lying in the tub relaxing, some of the best ideas come to mind. And it's truly a pain to get out of the tub and search for paper and pencil. Buy a supply of small tablets and put them in those locations.

◆ Incorporate a reasonable amount of structure into your life, not so much that you kill spontaneity, but enough to remember what comes next. So, get an appointment book or a calendar with large spaces to write in, and keep track of things you need to take care of. It doesn't just have to be places to go, but anything you need or want to do. When you get your book/calendar, sit down and fill in all the birthdays you want to remember. Draw a picture of a birthday cake or simply a candle. Do the same for other important family events or friends' special times that you want to remember. You might end up with the most exciting appointment book in town. Even better, of course, do all this using your newly acquired computer skills on your laptop.

◆ Give yourself cues about the matters you want to remember rather than relying solely on your unassisted memory. For example, let's say that you realize, as you're getting ready for bed, that you have to take your suit to the cleaners the next morning. To make sure you don't forget, put the suit right in front of the bedroom door.

◆ In a similar vein, whenever you find a task you want to remember to do, try to at least start it right away. That way, if you forget it, your memory will be jogged when you notice it half completed. As we discussed earlier, recognition is much easier than unaided recall. The renowned psychologist B. F. Skinner wrote of the "prosthetic environment" for older adults, and advised that they "rely on memoranda rather than memory." Among his many proactive suggestions was using timers to turn off appliances automatically; tape recorders to instantly capture ideas that might otherwise be quickly forgotten; and Post-it notes for items "to be remembered."

You may even come up with better solutions than we have, plus Chapter 5 is filled with ideas and techniques to help you in your commitment to solve your memory dilemmas. The important thing, however, is a strong desire and the commitment to start to do things that reduce your forgetting.

LEARNING MORE THAN YOU FORGET

You will have observed that certain people continue to be amazingly alert and appear to have remarkable memories well into old age. Partly, that is because they have assiduously exercised their minds, keeping their conductivity channels clear and hence their learning and remembering capacities in high gear.

However, there is a separate reason that some of these people appear to have such remarkable memories. An example is Brenda Adderly's husband's father, Walter Engel. He was a marvelously urbane and educated gentleman who, well into his eighties, regularly amazed people by his broad knowledge of everything from medieval architecture to the formula for PS. (For those of you who are interested, it is provided in the glossary at the end of this book.)

One day, Walter was visiting a new neighbor whom he had never met. Unbeknownst to him, she owned an impressive collection of twelfth-century ecclesiastical carvings of which she was enormously proud. As Walter entered her house, he could not fail to notice them beautifully hung and tastefully lighted on the walls of her large living room. "Very beautiful," he murmured. Then, pointing to one of the smaller pieces, he named the carver, an Italian monk unknown by anyone except the experts. "I've rarely seen his work in a private collection," he said.

Naturally, his hostess was astonished and delighted. "Oh," she gushed, "you are obviously a real connoisseur."

"Well, no." Walter shook his head truthfully. "It's just that I remember seeing some of his work in Rome quite a few years ago."

"Then you must have a marvelous memory," the lady praised.

"Not nearly as good as it used to be," Walter admitted modestly. "Twenty years ago, I would have remembered *all* your carvers' names."

The point is that, by most people's standards, Walter had a remarkable memory. But as he realized—and, at least on this occasion, was willing to acknowledge—his memory was actually no longer particularly impressive. It was just that he had such a large bank of information from which to draw that, even if he forgot most of what he knew, what remained was still so substantial that his memory *seemed* impressive.

A second advantage of exercising your mind to keep it nimble, then, is that in doing so you will add to your store of knowledge. If you do this assiduously, as people do who are enthusiastically wrapped up in their professions or their hobbies, you may be able to add to your pile of remembered information as fast as or faster than you forget what you already know. As a result, in a strange way, your memory, having more information stored in it, may be said to be improved even though your memory capacity may still be declining.

STEP 3

Protect Your Health, Eat a Healthy Diet and Add PS-Boosting Supplements

An appropriate diet can further enhance mental acuity and memory, adding to the effectiveness of PS, by adding foods to your diet that include natural sources of brain-boosting supplements. The right diet can optimize energy and ensure sound sleep patterns, making the brain more responsive and mentally alert.

A correctly balanced diet should contain a number of nutritional ingredients, especially antioxidants, known to be helpful for optimum mental and physical health. Thus, a correct diet can work together with a sound eating program to provide our bodies and our brains with the nutrients they need to be maximally effective. It can begin as soon as your next meal. A high intake of the primary vitamin antioxidants (see Chapter 7 for what they are) will help to protect against aging, and its concomitant loss of memory.

A free radical is a highly reactive chemical molecule that has lost one or more of its paired electrons. One group of writers calls it "a molecule wounded by exposure to life's nasties."[76] Its unpaired condition forces it to try to attract—actually "abduct" would be a more appropriate word—electrons from whole molecules, thus seriously damaging or destroying them. In this way, free radicals can damage basic genetic material, cell walls, and other cell structures. They can kill neurons and destroy neurotransmitters. Their production increases as time passes and we are exposed for more and more years to the impacts of such environmental factors as pollution, ultraviolet light, alcohol, tobacco smoke, and other environmental factors that catalyze free radical production. These free radicals are considered responsible for much of the normal aging process. The free radical theory of aging suggests that small but lifelong defects in protection against free radicals cause progressive tissue damage.[77]

In humans the most common free radicals are "activated" oxygen molecules, natural by-products of our metabolic process, as well as of the environmental factors mentioned above. As their name implies, antioxidants neutralize free radicals, and they do it by "filling up" their need for extra electrons.[78] So does PS, at least in the laboratory.

We'll talk more in Chapters 6 and 7 about how sound nutrition can help you achieve a wide awake, maximally effective state—but you may be surprised to learn that one of the most simple things you can do to help your memory is to drink sufficient water during the day. As we age, the total amount of our body fluids tends to decrease. This increases the sensitivity of our circulatory system to changes in water and salt levels. Lack of sufficient water, or dehydration, becomes much easier and can produce apathy, depression, and confusion, resulting in attention and memory difficulties.

STEP 4

Change Your Attitude Toward Stress

Stress ranks among the world's highest risk factors for bringing on all kinds of health problems.[79] In brief, stress is the body's response to change, whether pleasant or unpleasant. Like it or not, change occurs constantly. The real problem with stress, however, is the way we respond to it. Do we become aggressive or angry about it? Have we developed ways to cope with it that help us remain comfortable or restore balance?

In the hectic lives that many of us live, a certain amount of stress is unavoidable, but years of repeated stresses can lead to an array of health problems. For example, the cardiovascular system has been extensively studied and it has been conclusively shown that stress can lead to hypertension (high blood pressure), risk of coronary heart disease, and changes in blood clotting factors. These, in turn, lower our general feeling of well-being and tend to leave us lethargic and uninterested in doing much of anything at all, least of all exercising our memories with new learning inputs.

Like most of us, you've probably had the experience of being tense or nervous and having difficulty paying attention. This side effect of stress is not just psychological, however. Stress reduces circulation to the brain, starving brain cells of oxygen and nutrients. If the hippo-campus and the cortex sustain stress-related damage, memory and other cognitive functions are affected.

Clearly, then, elimination of stress—or, more practically, learning how to handle the stress we inevitably face so that it seems less aversive and does us less harm—is an important part of the memory cure. This will be discussed in more detail in chapter 8.

STEP *5*

Maintain Your Overall Health and Exercise Regularly

Many simple-to-treat health problems can adversely affect memory, as can many of the drugs prescribed to treat them, but it's not always a straightforward connection. Some drugs and diseases can affect short-term memory without affecting long-term memory, and vice versa.[80] Scientists have documented many health-related reasons for memory loss. Among them are fatigue, menopause, poor nutrition, vitamin deficiencies, drugs like tranquilizers and antihistamines, and any other diseases that subject us to acute discomfort.

Your doctor is the one best equipped to deal with these memory-related problems, and also can warn you of more serious problems, such as Alzheimer's disease, or help you minimize simpler ones such as hearing or visual problems. Since memory is a brain process that starts with sensory input, not being able to see or hear well, or the dulling of any of the other senses by injury, the use of medications, or other treatable disorders, can also reduce what you remember. Strategies that optimize overall health can prevent certain disorders, as well as the need for medication. Before embarking on any new health regimen, it is also important to check with your physician to assess your overall health and to discuss with him or her the specific steps you are considering.

Research in the 1980s suggested that activity level might be a major culprit in the memory loss of aging adults. Researchers had begun to criticize the fact that numerous studies in memory loss compared aging adults with younger adults. One group of researchers examined the results of memory tests of elderly residents living in a retirement community that provided them with an enriched environment, which included activities that kept them physically and cognitively active. They compared their responses with those of elderly persons who lived a more passive existence and with young college students. Sure enough, the "active" elderly scored as high on the particular tasks from this study as did the students.[81]

It was not clear from the research, however, whether the good memory results were due to the enriched environment or to the good health of the active persons, which allowed them to engage in a high level of activity. At least one group of researchers did find that elderly men who reported their health to be poor performed less well on a serial learning task, which required rehearsal/repetition, than individuals in the same age range who reported themselves to be in good health.[82]

More and more studies are being published that show

 MEMORY MOMENT _____

> " Life is all memory, except for the one present moment that goes by you so quick you hardly catch it going."
>
> —Tennessee Williams.

that paying attention to lifestyle factors (avoiding smoking, eating a low-fat diet high in fruits and vegetables, maintaining a moderate weight, exercising regularly) is necessary to maintain optimal health in our later years. The trick is to pay attention to healthful practices, yet not get obsessed about them.[83] Although we may not fully agree, Dr. Pelletier, author of *Sound Mind, Sound Body,*[84] even goes so far as to maintain that, in many fundamental respects, biologically there is little distinction between a healthy fifty-year-old and a healthy seventy-five-year-old.

One of the direct benefits of exercise is that it causes the release of the hormone neurotransmitter norepinephrine, which causes the brain to be more alert and also helps us to maintain a positive mood. Norepinephrine is crucial in helping carry memories from short-term storage into long-term storage.

Exercise increases circulation throughout the body. This means it also increases the amount of oxygen and glucose that the brain receives. It also helps stabilize blood sugar levels, which control mood and energy levels.

We shall discuss exercise in more detail in Chapter 9. For now, let us merely emphasize that this part of our memory boosting program is important to improve your memory—but vital to maintain yourself in good health for a long time to come. After all, wouldn't it be an ironic shame for you to maintain your memory in fine shape into your eighties and nineties, only to succumb to a body that fails you in your seventies due to a lack of exercise!

STEP 6

Maintain a Positive Attitude

If you believe you can improve your memory, you can. Researchers at Florida International University in

Miami found that your attitude toward intellectual aging correlates with how frequently you forget and how uncomfortable you are with forgetting. Because they think they're supposed to forget ("It's what happens when you get older"), older adults are not as uncomfortable with memory failures as younger adults, but they also rate themselves as more depressed.[85] We can wonder which comes first, their depression or their almost fatalistic acceptance.

The results of the Florida study are enhanced by a Mayo Clinic study. Researchers administered a series of memory and attitude scales to 294 people, aged 55 to 97 years, who originally had been assessed three years earlier. They found that emotional status was a better predictor of a person's subjective rating of his or her memory than was actual performance on a memory test.[86] Meaning, if you believe your memory is poor or fading, chances are you will act accordingly—for example, by not exercising it enough—and therefore worsen it until it is indeed as bad as you thought.

Rather, we urge you to be like the little blue engine in the children's story *The Little Engine That Could.* As you take your daily PS and increase its supply in your cell membranes, tell yourself, as the little engine did on its way to the top of the hill, that you *think* you can remember better than before and that you don't have to accept a lowered level of cognitive functioning. If you need a mantra for positive encouragement, each time you take your PS supplement, repeat like the little engine, "I think I can, I think I can."

Like that little engine, you *will* experience success.

BUYER BEWARE!

You'll need to be careful about making sure you are taking the level of PS required to be effective for improving AAMI. When we recommend a dosage of 300 milligrams of PS to start, and 100 milligrams for a sustaining level, what we mean is 300 milligrams and 100 milligrams of *PS*. However, PS is often sold as "PS complex," which includes other phospholipids in addition to the active ingredient, PS. Usually the "complex" is *only 20%* PS. Therefore, you will need 1,500 milligrams of the "complex" as a starting dose, and 500 milligrams as a sustaining dose. So don't be fooled if some manufacturer puts out a product with 100 milligrams of the "complex" at a low price. You would need 15 of those tablets to start, and 5 on a sustaining basis.

5

The Memory Maximizer

*Improving your recall for names, numbers,
faces, and lists*

◆

Remembering to take your medicine

◆

Bank those memories

◆

Don't forget the Internet

❖

In the course of history, there has been no shortage of
ideas for improving a weak memory. All too often,
those ideas have identified poor memory as a single problem that could be fixed with a single solution—some
fairly sensible, some quite outrageous. For instance, during the seventeenth century, people might be advised to
wear a cap made of beaverskin and/or to anoint their head
and spine monthly with drops of castor oil.[87] Would that
it were so simple!

Laying the Foundation

Four basic skills essential for learning to develop good
memory strategies are: intent, concentration/focus, confidence that you *can* remember what you intend to remember, and getting organized.

◆ **Intention.** If you don't have the intention or motivation to learn and practice memory techniques, you're
likely not going to do very well. Just reading this chapter
may give you some ideas that work, but most of them
require practice. Once you have mastered a particular

MEMORY MOMENT _____

FAMOUS FEATS OF MEMORY

The well-known orchestral conductor Arturo Toscanini had such poor vision that when he conducted he had to rely on his memory. He knew each note played by each instrument for 250 symphonies and 100 operas. Once when an orchestra member told Toscanini, then 19, that the lowest note on his bassoon was broken, Toscanini searched his memory and informed the musician that it was okay because that note didn't appear in any of the music they were playing that evening.

According to The Guinness Book of Records, on March 9–10, 1987, Hideaki Tomoyori of Yokohama, Japan, recited pi to 40,000 places, taking 17 hours and 21 minutes (including breaks of 4 hours, 15 minutes). Guinness doesn't say how long it took him to memorize the information in the first place.

In 1993, Dominic O'Brien of Great Britain memorized, with one look and only one mistake, a random sequence of 40 separate decks of cards that had been shuffled together, a total of 2,080 cards. How long, we wonder, had O'Brien been practicing his memory skills?

technique, you still need to practice. Say you've memorized a list. If you need to keep that list in memory for any length of time, you have to go over it mentally several times. You *must* practice.

◆ **Focus.** The basic foundation of all successful mental performance is the ability to focus and concentrate. Memory is a skill. The more you can focus or observe, the easier it is to add items to your memory and to recall them. Busy executives often report that sustained focus is the key to their business success.

Many of the gold-medal athletes interviewed after their performance at the 1998 Olympics in Nagano, Japan, remarked, "I just went out there and focused on my goal" (or "my technique," or "my performance"). Frequently, they also mentioned that they had fun during their performance, even though many were breathing heavily when they were interviewed or were clearly exhausted.

Consider how easy it is for you to concentrate on a movie you really enjoy. We've heard people say, "I really got into it and forgot the passage of time" with regard to a good book, an athletic event, or other enjoyable activities. For the most part, however, developing sustained focus and concentration requires expending effort—physical for movement activities, and the deliberate effort of will for mental activities. Consciously observing things you see and noticing the similarities and differences, paying attention to details, will in itself increase your ability to remember without any other special technique. You may also find that it will arouse your curiosity ("Why is this one made this way and that one made another way?" "How did you create that effect?") and set you on a path to discover new facts and develop new interests.

◆ **Confidence.** This is an extremely important factor in memory retention. If you worry about your ability to accomplish any of the exercises in this chapter, that worry can interfere with your learning the technique by overloading your processing system with anxious thoughts. Believe in yourself. Develop the idea that you can learn to remember better, and it's likely that you will.

At least one well-known memory researcher, who has conducted dozens of studies, suggests that memory training will not lead to lasting improvement in older adults who *believe* that age is the true cause for memory problems. Studies show that just having this belief will result in further deterioration of memory performance.[88] It is a self-fulfilling prophecy: "I'm going to forget things more and more because I'm getting old, and I do. There's nothing I can do about it; it's just what happens." If you have this notion, take a vow today to free yourself from this false perception.

Of course, this advice is easier to give than to accept. "How can I give myself conviction about something I don't believe?" you might reasonably ask. "If I could do that," a friend of ours pointed out, "I could believe in any impossible task. They'd lock me up as a crazy man— unless I inadvertently killed myself first by jumping out of a window because I knew I could fly."

The answer is that, if you are reading these words, you are obviously a rational person who is willing to base your belief on *facts*. And the fact is that you do not have to lose your memory. As we prove in this book, you can start reversing any memory decline from which you may be suffering right now (and the more thoroughly you delve into the research, the more certain you will be of the truth of that statement).

◆ **Organization.** The fourth factor that determines how much and how easily you remember is organization. Most of us have probably said at some time or another that we "have to get organized" or, more often, that it's something we'll "get around to" one of these days. It is one of the simplest ways to increase your memory. We're not talking about cleaning your basement, or taking a week to put everything in your house in a specific place. We're talking about changes that can be made in minutes, or sometimes seconds.

Many of the techniques in this chapter simply help

you organize, or reorganize, in a specific or unusual way, the material you want to remember. When the organization occurs solely in your mind, it is called "association" or linking.

Sometimes you organize not only your mind but your environment better. For example, if gathering and paying your bills is a task you find hard to remember, we suggest you develop a specific place where you always put your unpaid bills. Similarly, you can create a specific place where you always put your keys or your eyeglasses, or whatever it is you tend to lose most frequently. One colleague has a special pair of computer glasses, which she had to search for each time she sat down to work because she could never remember where she put them. She has finally solved this problem: now when she finishes for the day, she puts her glasses on the computer keyboard and, to reinforce this easily overlooked action, she says to herself, "Now I am putting my glasses on the keyboard." After doing that for several days—out loud at first, and now to herself—the acts and the words become such a routine that she probably couldn't forget them even if she wanted to! The result? Well, she hasn't misplaced her computer glasses since.

You're Never Too Old

Memory training can help prevent and correct forgetfulness at any age. Individuals who make the effort to challenge their brains make new neuronal connections through mental activity. They will, therefore, have less age-related memory loss than mental "couch potatoes." In this chapter we provide specific memory-training exercises to optimize your capacity to memorize material.

Use the exercises to earn a gold medal in your own "memory marathon" event.

As suggested by the interviews with Olympians, the exercises should be fun, but should also involve some effort. Unfortunately, as we've said before, memory doesn't work like a muscle. You can't exercise your way to a stronger or perfect memory no matter how many of the Memory Maximizer exercises you use. By using these techniques, however, you can develop, discover, and practice memory skills that work particularly well for enhancing your memory. You can improve your memory technique.

Be prepared to experience some anxiety, nervousness, or concern as you practice your new skills. It's to be expected. Psychologist Jerome Kagan tells us that the "key tension" in every problem we encounter is that our first reaction is to use the knowledge and abilities that have worked for us in the past. Pitted against that is the awareness that, in this case, the "old ways" are no longer adequate and must be altered. We have to be able to "hang in there"—to persevere—long enough to overcome this tension.[89]

Because not everyone enjoys the same thing, the Memory Maximizer plan includes all of the following:

◆ word games, mind teasers, and crossword puzzles
◆ mnemonic devices
◆ imagery and visualization techniques
◆ association techniques
◆ memorization challenges
◆ exercises to improve the recall of names, numbers, faces, and lists

One word of warning: Don't just participate in the exercises you know you enjoy, or already know how to do.

Face the "key tension." Train those "little gray cells" by practicing techniques that are a little hard for you and require a little more focus and concentration.

Styles of Creating Memories

We develop our information about the world and create our memories through our five senses. Most of us rely primarily on one of three sensory information systems—visual, auditory, and, to a lesser degree, tactile (i.e., sense of touch)—rather than all five. This means that generally we have learned to rely on taking in and learning information about the world primarily through our eyes, ears, and also through touch. The other senses—smell and taste—can also contribute to memories, but not as heavily, and, of course, no one uses one of these styles of learning exclusively.

The human brain evolved to encode and interpret all of the complex stimuli received by our senses, so the more senses you can activate to learn a situation, the more easily you will be able to learn and recall it. By activating senses other than your usually dominant visual and auditory ones and creating imaginary images, you will be using more of your mental resources than just language. So, for example, when you want to remember something like a phone number, the visual image is how you see the number on your telephone keypad. Saying the number aloud activates your auditory memory, and punching the number in serves as a kinesthetic aid. If you just want to remember and don't want to reach the number, then imagine punching out the number in your mind, moving your fingers as you do so, or actually placing them on the appropriate buttons on your phone.

◆ **Characteristics of Visual Learners.** About 65

percent of us are visual learners and remember best if we can see written information or take notes, whether or not we keep the material. Even if you are not a visual learner, writing down what you want to remember forces you to focus your attention on it, at least for a few moments, and calls upon your kinesthetic senses to assist you.

The techniques in this chapter that employ writing things down, drawing diagrams, or visualizing pictures will appeal most to visual learners. However, some people may find that they are less able to see mental images than they could when they were younger, especially if they have gotten away from the habit of developing images. If this applies to you, practicing those techniques will be especially helpful. (Separately, you may also want to practice looking at a picture or diagram, and then, without looking, trying to visualize it as accurately as possible. You will soon find much of your old visual memory returning.)

Writing lists of things you have to do has the double advantage of focusing your attention and providing both visual and motor cues (good for kinesthetic learners and for engaging more than one sensory system). Hence, some of the simplest things you can do to make your memory more efficient is to use an appointment book or calendar, keep a list of things you want to do, and put numbers by the items to indicate the order of priority or importance. Research shows that list-making significantly improves the performance of older adults on recall tasks, and that organizing their lists improves the recall of both young and old "list-makers" more than applies to those who did not organize their lists.[90] And, of course, a list has the actual advantage that, if you do forget, the list is there to remind you!

There's nothing wrong with using external memory

aids. Most of us at some time or another need a cue to remind us of what we're supposed to do.

◆ **Kinesthetic Learners.** About 15 percent of the population learn and remember best if they can connect the situation with movement. Top-notch athletes usually have good kinesthetic memory. Not only can they remember complex muscle movements, but research has shown that by creating images in their mind, they can activate their muscles and the area of the brain that coordinates them, perfect required movements, and even practice new ones by creating images in their minds.

Those who rely on kinesthetic learning and remembering (i.e., who tend to enjoy learning by imitating and practicing movement) will do so most effectively through exercises that emphasize both the feeling of movement and movement itself. A popular technique in recent years athletes use to perfect their skill is to mentally picture themselves moving through all of the actions of their particular sport, or that part of the sport they want to enhance, as if they were watching themselves in a movie. Scans of the brain using positron emission tomography (PET scans) show that imagined activity stimulates the same parts of the brain as real activity.

◆ **Talk to Yourself.** Auditory learners, about 20 percent of us, relate most effectively to the spoken word and will learn and remember best those things that involve sound or that they can repeat aloud. Students who are highly auditory in their learning skills often find they remember better if they read their assignments or notes aloud and recite the facts they need to remember for tests. The more drama they can bring into their readings, i.e., the more interesting they are to listen to, the better they will remember.

If you frequently find yourself forgetting whether you

locked the front door, unplugged the iron, or turned off the computer, remind yourself out loud. As you lock the door, say "Now I've locked the door," or "Now I'm locking the door, and I won't need to check it again." Janet Fogler, a social worker and coauthor of *Improving Your Memory: How to Remember What You're Starting to Forget,* says that hearing your own voice confirming an action is remarkably effective in helping you remember.[91] But don't mumble as you speak. The more authority you put into your voice, the more likely you are to remember it, just as would apply if someone else were speaking to you.

Even for predominantly visual learners, talking over something you want to remember with friends, or telling it as a story, is an excellent way to help make a memory stick. Your memory improves as you tell and retell the event. Hearing yourself say it out loud improves memory whether or not someone else is around.

Setting a timer to remind you to do something is a tried-and-true technique for using sound to help you remember something. A friend of ours who works at home and tends to get involved in her work and forget other things sets a timer on her desk to ring when she needs to move the garden hose, or heat the oven for dinner. That way she knows she can immerse herself in her work without mental interruption.

MOVE IT, DON'T LOSE IT

That same friend uses another good memory technique to remind herself to take care of certain things: she changes something in her home or office so that she remembers it. For instance, if she needs to make an important phone call on a particular day, she moves the telephone from her desk to the floor in front of her office door. It's the old tie-a-string-around-your-finger technique, only on a larger scale. We've heard a lot about the string technique and wonder if anyone still uses it, but the principle is sound. Turn a ring around or switch it from one hand to the other to remind you of something that needs to be done.

Put a note in your cereal bowl, or on your computer, to remind you to do something first thing in the day. Or keep a basket by the door to place things you have to take with you the next day, or that have to be transported to the office from home or vice versa.

Word Games, Mind Teasers, and Crossword Puzzles

Although crossword puzzles are a great way to keep your intellect alive and to learn new vocabulary, we know many of you don't like doing crossword puzzles. If you are one of those people, then this section will give you some additional ideas for building your brainpower and enhancing your memory. Participating in word games and mind teasers doesn't so much improve your memory as challenge your brain, keeping neurons active. They are the enriched environment that keep those dendrites branching. There are many books on the market that contain puzzles and problems designed to do just that. A challenge a day keeps the muddle away!

◆ **Stretch, Stretch, Stretch Your Imagination.** Sitting where you are, look at some object in the room and imagine how it would look if you were standing behind it, at either side of it, floating above it. This is an excellent mind-stretcher when you are looking at photographs in a book or magazine. Imagine how the scene would look from different positions or imagine how it would look if photographed in a different season—covered with snow or ice, or bathed in sunlight.

The mother of a three-year-old told us how she took her son to her office on the thirtieth floor of a New York skyscraper. Looking out of the window, she pointed at the traffic below. "Look at all the toy cars," she said. The child was delighted. But a little later when they left the building, the boy burst into tears.

"What's the matter?" the mother asked.

"I want the toy cars," the boy sobbed, "and they're all gone!"

If we could learn to change our perspective as easily as we could when we were five-year-olds, we'd be able to exercise our minds so vigorously that we'd probably never lose our memories at all!

◆ **Illustrate a Poem.** You are an artist and you have been given the assignment to illustrate a particular poem of your choice. Don't worry about your artistic abilities; you are going to do this in your imagination. You will paint with your mind's eye, although you may actually draw or paint if you prefer.

Read a poem of your choice, and take the time to imagine what each line would look like in your painting or photography. If you're not sure where to start, try William Blake: "Tyger, tyger burning bright" practically illustrates itself! (Blake said he spelled it like that because it was a very special tiger!) Illustrating a poem will exercise your visual imagination in ways you never thought of. And, of course, it will help you remember the poem. (You do remember "Tyger, tyger burning bright." Now try "In the forests of the night." Illustrate that and see if you can ever forget it!)

◆ **Learn New Words.** There is a word-a-day calendar on the market that introduces you to a new word each day. If one word each day is too much for you, then just learn two words each week and commit them to memory. Learn about the roots and derivations of foreign or complex words. Use your new words as soon as you can in a conversation or in a letter. Try creating a sentence or phrase with the new word in it to help you remember the meaning and context of the new word.

◆ **Activate Those Neurons.** Put together a jigsaw puzzle or get a book of mazes and work your way through them. Get a word-scramble book with lines of scrambled words and find the original words in each line. Each of these activities keeps the neurons in different parts of your brain active. For instance, the scrambled words below have all been used in this book. What are they? (Answers are at the end of the chapter.)

> r i b a n
>
> y s n s p e a
>
> m y r o e m
>
> t r o f i n g t e g

To help you recall words you rarely use more quickly try this exercise: Write out your name and place it at the top of a piece of paper. Using a word that begins with each letter in your name in order, write yourself a telegram. For instance, Tom Crook might write himself a message that reads: "The old man called. Running overtime. Obey Karen." Then try to make a full sentence of it: "The old man calls regularly only on Kate." Is it easier if you don't have to use the letters in order? Find out. Write your own telegram to Tom, or to yourself. Do it as fast as you can. Try making another sentence quickly: "To ordinary men, crying risks overloading our karma." Hmm!

◆ **Think of New Solutions.** This is the kind of problem that is often included on I.Q. tests. Can you solve it?

A boy's mother sends him to the river, telling him to bring back exactly one cup of water. She gives him a four-cup can and a three-cup can and tells him to bring back exactly one cup using nothing but the two cans. How can the boy bring back one cup?

Now that you have that one figured out (the answer is at the end of the chapter), solve the problem using an eight-cup can and a five-cup can to get 11 cups. This boy's mother is very demanding, but she wants him to grow up using his brain, so in the next trip, she sends him to the river to bring back three cups, using only a four-cup can and a nine-cup can.

Draw a two-inch line on a piece of paper. Without changing the line in any way (or folding the paper—we've already thought of that), make the line shorter.

Mnemonic Devices

According to Greek mythology it was Mnemosyne (NEE-mos-en-NEE), the Greek goddess of memory and mother of the Muses, who gave us our ability to remember. She herself knew everything, past, present, and future. Linguists did take her name to form the word "mnemonics" (NEE-mon-icks, the first m being silent), various strategies for helping us organize and remember information by linking items together to help you remember. During medieval times mnemonic techniques were considered so powerful that they were classified among the "magic arts."[92] In the seventeenth century, they were used by famous philosophers such as Francis Bacon and Wilhelm Leibniz as a way of organizing knowledge.

The Roman orator Cicero informed us about the first

mnemonic technique. His story says that around 500 B.C., Scopas, a nobleman of Thessaly, gave a banquet to celebrate a wrestling victory, and hired the poet Simonides of Ceos to chant a lyric poem in Scopas's honor. Simonides made a bad decision and included a passage praising the twin gods Castor and Pollux. Angered, Scopas decided to pay Simonides only half the sum agreed on and sarcastically informed Simonides that he could collect the rest from Castor and Pollux.

When given a message that two young men were waiting to see him, Simonides left the banquet hall but found no one. While he was outside, the roof of the hall fell in and crushed all the guests. Cicero suggests that the two young men were Castor and Pollux, paying their debt.

In remembering where the guests had been sitting, Simonides helped relatives identify their dead. From this experience, he devised the first known visual imagery system of mnemonics, variations of which are used to this day. Simonides imagined a room—a "memory palace"—in which he "placed" items he wanted to remember in special locations. Then when he wanted to recall those items, he needed only to use his mind's eye to "look" at the appropriate place in the room. Simonides' technique has come to be called the Loci (LOW-kigh) technique. The word *loci* is the plural of the Greek word *locus,* which means "place" or "location."

◆ **Creating a Memory Palace.** The Loci technique is a good one for remembering the main points of a speech or presentation. In fact, it was the way Greek and Roman orators remembered and presented long speeches without notes. Think of a house or building you know well. Place an image representing the first point of your speech in the entryway of the house. As you continue in an orderly procession through the house, place an image representing your second, third, and continuing points in those rooms you pass through. When you get ready to make your presentation, you simply have to picture yourself walking through the house where you will see, in their correct order, images representing the points you want to make.

◆ **Filling Your Palace.** If you choose to use the "memory palace" to help you remember items, you can use your own house or a house you make up in your imagination. Decorate each room with furniture, windows, etc. Create the images you want to remember and put them in various places in the room, on the furniture, in the windows. Associate them with whatever items you have placed in the room. In the beginning, don't place more than four or five images in any one room in the house. Not crowding the room with images helps memory, although as you get more skilled with the technique, you will be more able to increase the number of images in each room. Also, it is helpful to use images that employ unusual colors or objects, or ones that are interesting, unusual, or interactive.[93]

If you play golf, use a golf course that you are most familiar with. You now have 36 locations (18 tees and 18 greens) on which you can place items you need to remember or the points you want to make in a presentation. As you give that fabulous "extemporaneous" speech, you are, in fact, enjoying a stroll through the golf course.

When college freshmen in a "study skills" course were taught the Loci method to remember the main ideas in a prose passage, they recalled 50 percent more ideas from a 2,200-word passage than did students taught traditional study skills.[94]

You don't have to be a student memorizing material for an examination to benefit from the Loci method. Several research studies have demonstrated that it is also an excellent technique for helping older adults remember a grocery list.[95] Suppose you need to go to the market to buy paper towels, milk, apples, coffee, cat food, celery, and eggs. Close your eyes now and try to remember the list before you read on.

Using the Loci technique, you can imagine paper towels rolled out along the length of your front walk. When you reach the front door, a half-dozen milk bottles sit beside it. As you enter the living room, you check one of your locations—the desk beside the window—and find that the top of it is empty except for one giant apple. Noticing the rug on the floor, you see that someone has spilled coffee grounds on it. Checking another location—your cozy chair—you see that it is filled with hungry cats. Cats lounging on it, hanging from it, peeking out from under it. As you look out the window, you observe a tree that is made from the stalks of a giant bunch of celery. The tips of the celery drape downward like a weeping willow and sitting in the middle of the tree is a nest of brilliantly colored Easter eggs.

If you are an auditory learner, enhance the images in a house by having them make sounds. Hear the crunch of the apple and celery, the cats meowing, the eggs cracking. If you are primarily a kinesthetic learner, imagine scenes that are in action or imagine performing actions yourself, and even move your body in the actions you create, to help you lock in what you want to remember. Roll out the paper towels, have the milk bottles dancing or swaying, have an apple tree growing apples.

◆ **Organizing by Numbers or Categories.** If you associate what you need to remember with a number or sequence, it often helps your memory to become more efficient. For instance, before Jane goes out to run errands, she mentally makes a list of what she needs, assigning specific numbers to each errand. Sometimes she simply uses the numbers alone, knowing, for instance, that she has five things to accomplish. Now, she doesn't always remember them in order, but one-by-one she recalls them until she has accomplished all five.

She might improve her memory by organizing her tasks by category. Suppose she has five tasks she needs to do before she and her husband can go away for the weekend: buy cat food, call the neighbor to be sure she feeds the cats, gather maps from the auto club, pick up her coat from the cleaners, and buy suntan lotion. She might organize her tasks this way:

> Grocery—2
> Cats—1
> Pickup—2

Then she repeats several times what these organizing cues actually refer to, helping to anchor them in her memory.

◆ **Use Rhymes or Sentences to Improve Memory.** Rhymes and simple sentences are a handy form of mnemonic, one of the reasons being that a stronger relationship exists between the words in a sentence than between a list of words. Probably every kid who ever had a music lesson remembers being taught to remember the lines of the G-clef with the sentence Every Good Boy Does Fine, e-g-b-d-f. And that the spaces between the lines spell FACE. Easier for a budding musician than stalling while you quickly recite to yourself the whole sequence of e-f-g-a-b-c-d-e-f before you can tell your teacher the line or space a note was placed on.

Baby or amateur astronomers may have been taught, as we were in college, to remember the order of the nine

planets then known in the solar system with the sentence
My Very Earnest Mother Just Served Us Nine Pickles:
Mercury, Venus, Earth, Mars, Jupiter, Saturn, Uranus,
Neptune, Pluto.

And for budding geographers, the Great Lakes spell
HOMES: Huron, Ontario, Michigan, Erie, and Superior.

Rhymes make material easier to learn. Experts think
this is because when a list of words is recalled, words
that rhyme tend to be recalled together, plus the fact that
other words that rhyme with a word may be effective cues
to help recall it.[96] Many of us still use two popular rhyming mnemonic techniques to figure out how many days
there are in a month:

> Thirty days hath September,
> April, June, and November.
> All the rest have 31,
> save February which has 28
> (except in leap year, when it has 29).

If you weren't good at rhymes, however, then there
was the mnemonic trick of counting on your knuckles
and the spaces or valleys in between. The first knuckle is
January, and has 31 days. The valley next to it is February (28 days, the exception). Next knuckle, March, 31
days. And so on. When you reach the last knuckle, you
start over. It turns out to be July, 31 days. Then you begin
again, the first knuckle becomes August, also 31. After
that, the valley is September, 30 days. And the sequence
holds. Imagine that! How did our smart knuckles know?

Songs with catchy rhymes or rhythm are also good
memory aids. Remember your child singing that rhyming
commercial over and over until you longed to send her
off to another planet? If you saw the movie *The Sound of
Music*, no doubt you remember how Julie Andrews

taught the Von Trapp children to remember the names of the musical scale with a song that begins:

> Doe, a deer, a female deer,
> Ray, a drop of golden sun . . .

If you saw the movie and heard the song, we bet you can finish it, and with it never forget the note sequence, "do, re, me, fa, so, la, ti, do."

Recent theories of how the brain works influence the whole question of whether memories are "true" or "false." A large body of research has shown that memories are often somewhat distorted. Recovered memories may be particularly unreliable, especially in borderline patients who may have had a distorted perception of the interpersonal events to begin with.[97]

According to the research of Dr. Gerald Edelman, the brain chooses images, sounds, and other sensations and interpretations registered in the past and then combines them to produce what we call a memory. This "memory" may be an accurate depiction of something that happened, but it can just as easily be a personal creation, using information from various incidents.[98]

It's very likely that in trauma, when emotions and sensations are intense—and may even be on overload—that the actual memory of the experience is fragmented. Consequently, only fragments of a remembered traumatic event are likely to be entirely accurate when they are reremembered, while other parts may be derived from different experiences as the aroused nervous system searches around and tries to comprehend the re-aroused emotion.

Cognitive psychologist Craig Barclay asked college students to keep a diary in which they recorded things that happened to them just after they occurred (actual memories). Dr. Barclay collected the diaries and subsequently tested the students' memories for these events at delays ranging from several months to two years. Sometimes he showed them a printed version of an actual diary and asked them if this was exactly what they had written down. Other times the descriptions were changed in various respects, like adding that a person had hunted for a gift in ten stores before giving up, when, in fact, she had never written that in her diary. As time passed, students increasingly agreed that the changed descriptions (false memories) were exactly what they had written down earlier.[99]

Naturally, then, as people age, more and more false memories of long-past facts will occur. While this does not mean that, in theory, older people's memories of immediate facts will necessarily be worse, it does suggest that older people's memories will be more confused by incorrectly remembered data. Therefore, they are more likely to confuse all memory, distant or fairly recent. (For example, if you incorrectly remember that San Diego is north of San Francisco, you will probably also misremember its climatic conditions. Your current memory will be confused by incorrect earlier information.)

Jog Your Memory

Have you ever had the experience of going from one room to another with the intention of doing something specific, only to find that when you got into the second room, you couldn't remember why you went there? Returning immediately to the first room where the thought occurred, or engaging in the activity you were doing when you originally had the thought, often helps you to recover it. That is because it has become associated with the room or with what you were doing at the time you thought of it. This is why witnesses to an accident or crime are sometimes interviewed, or re-interviewed, at the scene of the occurrence. If they are taken back there they are better able to remember the details of what they saw than they could when they were away from the scene.

There are many ways of jogging your memory, of course, as we have discussed elsewhere. But they all boil down to a simple principle: if you have trouble remembering a whole scenario or piece of learning, concentrate instead on a single bit of the subject, preferably a bit that ties into something you already know. Then remembering that bit will bring back the entire memory.

Chunking

Mathematician A. C. Aitken, a professor at Edinburgh University, could recall the first thousand decimal places of pi, the symbol denoting the ratio of a circle's circumference to its diameter. He did this by arranging the digits in a certain pattern or "chunk" of numbers, and then reading them over in a certain rhythm. An interesting technique for which you can probably find even more probable uses!

You will remember from an earlier chapter that "chunking," or breaking down long lists of information into shorter bunches, is a basic technique both for short-term memory improvement and for transferring material we want to remember from short-term to long-term memory. By grouping or organizing what we want to remember into larger and larger chunks, we increase the amount of material we can retain. The important point here is not that this is merely a mnemonic trick, but that it is a form of what communication theorists call "recoding." According to Dr. George A. Miller, who first recognized it, chunking is an "extremely powerful weapon for increasing the amount of information that we can deal with."[100] It's no accident that the telephone company breaks long-distance ten-digit numbers into three chunks of three, three, and four digits.

Whenever you need to remember a long list of apparently isolated facts, numbers, or letters, break them into chunks. Thus the series 366890467902476 now becomes five chunks: 366-890-467-902-476. Time yourself on how long it takes you to remember and write down these five chunks. Then practice breaking the following series into chunks and memorizing them:

254783571
AKGYWTQIO
469257981379
WPALQYRXAJKS

Now see how you do on a span of 15 digits or letters (hint: chunk the digits into three groups of five each):

291837640838562
KQOEPSRITMXUAFU

Imagery and Visualization Techniques

As we progress through life, most of us are discouraged from using our spontaneous, imaginative behavior. "Be serious," parents and others say to us. "Stop making things up." We're here to tell you that your imaginative ability is an important feature in increasing your memory skills. Using your imagination to create an image is one kind of mnemonic that can help you remember lists (of words or activities) instead of memorizing them.

For example, if you want to remember the words cat, chicken, television, lamp, you could create a picture in your mind of a cat chasing a chicken. Both jump onto the television and knock over the lamp, which goes crashing. You've used your imagination to activate not only language, but visual, kinesthetic (action), and auditory (sound) senses.

Have fun with your memory by making your images humorous. Funny or peculiar things are easier to remember than those that are not. Similarly, positive, pleasant images are generally easier to remember. Unless you are depressed, the brain tends to block out unpleasant imagery. Maybe you change the image above to a cat and a chicken, arm-in-wing, sitting in front of a television, trying to figure out how to turn off the lamp. Go on, make a unique image of your own with those four words. How can you use this technique for more practical things?

◆ **Remembering Your Grocery List.** Say you need to pick up several items at the grocery store: bath soap, milk, lightbulbs, and toothpaste. What can *you* do with that? Imagine yourself as a model in a television commercial for soap. You are sitting in a tub full of milk (because the soap keeps your skin as soft as a milk bath), holding up a bar of soap in a brilliant blue wrapper, and smiling like crazy with a mouthful of bright, shiny teeth. Your smile is so bright and dazzling that it shatters the lightbulbs in the lamps being used to film the commercial. Exaggeration of size, shape, speed, sound, and taste will all help to make the images in your scenes more memorable.

◆ **Remembering Your Appointments.** Now, make up an entertaining image for three, four, or five things you need to do tomorrow. For instance, Brenda Adderly needs to meet with her editor at 9 A.M. tomorrow, go to the library to pick up some research, and drop off a pair of shoes to be repaired. Before you read further, take a moment to consider what scene you can come up with to help her (and you) remember these appointments.

◆ **Color Makes Memory Easier.** Adding vivid color to an image makes it easier to remember than if it is drab or dull. Fill your imagination with brilliant purples and school bus yellows to help trigger your memory. Exaggeration of size ("an elephantine sofa") or number ("dozens of milk cartons") also improves memory.

Visualization is a good technique to remember items you need to buy at the grocery store, your schedule for the day, the name of a movie you want to see, the route from one place to another. If you can take the time to make a meaningful picture of what you want to remember, and fill it with items that involve as many of your senses as you can, you are more likely to remember it.

Association Techniques

New information is more easily transformed into long-term information by connecting it with other well-known and/or relevant information that already exists in long-term memory. The more associations you can make, the better something is remembered. Also, the more effort you put into creating associations, the more likely you are to recall it.

Association techniques are a form of mnemonics where you link things you want to remember with things you already know. One form of association is to connect one object with another. Think you've never done it? Think again. In one of its most simple but effective associations, hundreds of elementary school children have been taught to spell p*ie*ce correctly by linking it with p*ie*, a piece of pie. Associate the new word (piece) with an easier word we already know how to spell (pie), and, voilà, we never again have to ask whether piece is spelled with an "i before e" or "e before i." (Actually you can remember the same information, plus how to spell ceiling, with a short rhyme: "i" before "e" except after "c.")

Can you draw the correct shape of France or Germany from memory? Probably not, but we're willing to bet that you will come fairly close to drawing the shape of Italy because you've likely been taught, as we were, to remember that it resembles a boot. We learned by associating or linking the new shape (Italy) with something we already knew (boot).

Linking lets us remember more. We are forever grateful to the teacher who taught us that when we were in caves we could know stalactites (with a "c") because they grow from the ceiling while stalagmites grow from the ground. You can remember the difference in spelling and definition between stationery and stationary by knowing that an envelope (full of e's) is a piece of stationery.

Another form of association is to have two objects placed on each other in some way. For instance, sometimes instead of just remembering the number of errands she has to accomplish, Brenda finds it more fun and helpful to connect an unusual scene to each of the errands she needs to run. So when she needs to go to the market to get cat food, and to the dry cleaners to fetch her coat, she creates a vision of her two cats sitting on her coat and getting it full of hairs. Since that's probably what happened, she's unlikely to forget her vision—or her errands. Similarly, if you need to be reminded that the first thing you need to do when you get home is to invite friends for dinner, you might visualize an oval-shaped table filled with exotic foods to remind you to plan the dinner party.

People who are more kinesthetically oriented will find it easier to remember things or events if they are—or appear to be—in motion. Thus, to remember two images, they might imagine them interacting in some way, like merging together, wrapping around each other, or actively rotating or dancing around each other.

The Russian mnemonist Shereshevskii seemed to have no limit to the material he could memorize. The eminent neuropsychologist Alexander Romanovich Luria, who studied Shereshevskii extensively, discovered that his skill came from the fact that something he saw or heard with one sense automatically evoked an image in another, an ability called synesthesia.[101] For instance, when he was presented with a tone that had a pitch of 2,000 cycles per second, he remarked that it looked like fireworks tinged with a pink-red hue, felt rough, and had an ugly taste. He remembered numbers by experiencing them as shapes and colors, or as resembling people with definite personality characteristics (a "high-spirited woman"). Before you begin to envy or wish for Shereshevskii's ability, you should also know that he was plagued by the amount of incessant, useless recollections he had for trivial information and events. When he read or listened to a story, he recalled endless details but had little overall understanding of what he had read or heard. Shereshevskii also had great difficulty grasping abstract concepts.[102]

Like Shereshevskii, Rajan Mahadevan had an exceptional memory for lists of digits. When he was instructed to remember the position and orientation of 48 images of common objects (memory for spatial relations), however, his accuracy for judging whether position and orientation had changed when the images were shown in a different sequence was lower than that of eight "control" subjects for both judgments.[103] Alas, neither Shereshevskii nor Mahadevan had that elusive "perfect memory" either.

Memorization Challenges

◆ **Concentration: A Memory Game.** One good game for improving your memory is a "home version" of the popular television game *Concentration.* You can play it alone or with a partner, for as short or as long a time as you like, and you can make it as easy or as hard as you want. All it requires is a regular deck of 52 playing cards.

The basics of the game go like this. Shuffle your deck of cards and lay them out facedown in a convenient pattern (more about that later). Then turn one card faceup, memorize or make a mental note of what that card is, say a red king, or a black three, and its position, and return it to its facedown position. Choose a second card to turn over. If it is a match to the card you previously turned over, and you remember where that first card was, turn it over. You now have a pair, which you can remove from the table. If you have no match, return both cards to their original facedown position and start again, selecting another card to turn faceup. If this card matches one of the cards you have previously turned up, you need to remember where that card is, and turn it over, creating a matched pair that you can collect as your reward. Continue selecting pairs until all the cards are removed.

A two-player game using any number of cards can be great fun. Flip a coin to see who goes first. The player with the most pairs at the end of the game wins. You can make the game more challenging by setting a time limit, but don't get so concerned with the time that you forget to have fun.

The game is not as easy as it seems at first glance, and there are many variations to give you a lot of practice. You can change the number of cards used to go progressively from an easy game to a more difficult one. An easy way to play is to match *any color king* (or other denomination) with any other king. You then have three other possibilities for a match. To make the game more difficult, you can change the rules to require that the kings, or other denomination, must be opposite colors—or the same color—to be a match. You then have only one possibility. Even changing the pattern of the layout can make the game as challenging or as easy as you want it to be.

Here are some variations to make the game easier or harder:

1 A short game of 10 cards, five matching pairs, makes for a fast and interesting game, and requires a smaller area (about 8″ × 13″) than using a full deck. You could sort the cards so this "deck" has pairs of mixed colors or pairs of the same color to match. To complicate it, choose the pairs such that a red king must be matched with a black king, while a red 10 is to be matched with another red 10.

2 Use a 20-card "deck" and include only cards from ace (one) to 10 or, for variety, from five to king. Again, match for same color or opposite colors. Probably you would want to lay out this group of cards in four lines of five cards each, using an area

approximately 13″ by 15″. Having a friend choose the cards can add some diversity and unexpected challenge. It also gives you a chance to set up the deck for your friend for his or her next game.

3 If you create a 26-card "deck," you could use two suits (matching for the same color will be harder; matching opposite colors easier). Use a four-line layout with three lines of seven cards and one line of five cards. The area would cover about 15″ by 18″.

4 To use a full deck of 52 cards (or 54 with the jokers), you'll need a space about 24″ by 28″. One way to lay the cards out is with six rows, consisting of five rows of 10 cards each, with an extra row of two or four cards if you use the jokers.

◆ **Television as a Memory Booster.** Generally, we do not advocate watching much television. It tends to be more soporific than challenging. However, if you cannot do without your favorite sitcom or soap opera (and who among us can?), then you can still watch, have some fun with a friend or family member, *and* increase your observational skills at the same time. All you do is, before you watch your next television show, make a list of, say, a dozen questions that will test your observational powers and your memory. For example: "What are the names of the characters in the show"; "How many different locations are shown"; "What was the furniture in the room"; "What car models were shown"? Then, after the show, see how well you can answer your list. Of course, you can play this game alone, too. But if you do it with a friend, the best rememberer is the winner. A little competition always spices things up.

Improving Your Recall for Names, Numbers, Faces, and Lists

In "Your Shrinking Brain," a segment that aired on the television show *20/20* on January 9, 1998, Dr. Cynthia Green, who teaches a course in memory enhancement at Mt. Sinai Medical Center in New York, informed viewers that the foremost complaint of people as they grow older was the inability to remember names. On the other hand, sometimes a shrinking memory for names is the stuff of poets, as "commemorated" by the nineteenth-century poet Swinburne when he wrote:

> And the best and the worst of this is
> That neither is most to blame,
> If you have forgotten my kisses
> And I have forgotten your name.[104]

In spite of the practicalities of learning to remember names better, little research was done on it until the mid-1970s. Partly because they are so unusual or not as common as other words, names are harder to remember than, say, a list of words to remind you of errands.[105] Research conducted in 1997 indicates that memory for names and faces occurs partially in different brain systems.[106] Here are some proven techniques you can use to help you remember people to whom you have been introduced:

◆ **Use Distinctive Facial Features.** Where a name fits easily into a sentence, that is a good way of remembering the name. You won't forget the name "Will Patton" if you create the sentence "Will Patton conquer Italy?" However, relatively few names lend themselves to sentences. Therefore, a more widely useful technique is to identify a prominent or distinctive feature of the person's face (bushy or white eyebrows, a mole on the cheek), or a behavior pattern, smiling, frowning, or eating noisily, and connect that feature or characteristic with the name. Then when you want to recall a person's name, search your memory for the identifying feature. Even a complicated name—Gloria Feltenstein, for example—would be remembered by recalling that she has *glorious* skin as smooth as *felt* and served you beer in a *stein.*

◆ **Curiosity Helps Memory for Names.** For unusual names, it helps to immediately repeat it out loud to make sure you have it correctly and to program your memory by adding the phrase "that is an unusual name." In fact, it helps to remember any name more effectively if you make certain you get the name correct in the first place. If it is an unusual name, ask about it. Is it a special family name? What is the country of origin? During the ensuing conversation with the person, use the name at least twice, and more if you can. This reinforces your concentration. Always take time to have some conversation, if you can, before meeting someone else and having to learn a new name, since spacing introductions allows you time to make good associations to the name or face, and specific items in the conversation may also help to fix the name more firmly in your mind. Remember that one of the memory "interferers" we discussed in chapter 2 is that new information pushes out similar prior information. Therefore, try to make each new piece of data as different from prior pieces as possible.

◆ **Silly Pictures.** Another way to remember complicated names is to build a silly picture that will connect your memory with the person's name. You might help yourself remember Brenda Adderly's name by imagining a hot, sunny day and a field full of snakes (*adders*) sunning themselves as, understandably, Brenda quickly

*lea*ves the field. It helps the scene if you know what
Brenda looks like, so that you can visualize her as she
rushes away (see the photo on the book jacket).

If snakes aren't your thing, you might visualize the
same field, but this time it is full of people adding.
They're using giant adding machines and as they look at
the screens of their adding machines, what do you think
they see? Yes. Brenda's face. The rule here is that if you
can make mental fun of a name, it will be easier for you
to remember it.

If you meet several people at a party or meeting, when
it is over, mentally rehearse the names and faces again,
especially if there is a chance you are going to see them
again socially or professionally. Recall where in the
room you met them.

Some research shows that faces that you regard as
"distinctive" or memorable, or that you can make distinctive in some way in your own perception or in your
mind's eye (with imagination), coupled with the belief
that you will remember the face, enhance the ability to
remember faces.[107]

Another study shows that it is easier to remember both
faces and names if you can connect the person's occupation with the face/name.[108] Hence, when you are meeting
someone, taking the time to chat with that person long
enough to find out his or her occupation may give you a
memory advantage.

◆ **Associating the Name with Someone You Know.**
This is very effective if the new name you are trying to
memorize is the same as, or even similar to, another
name that you are unlikely to forget. Brenda's husband
likes to refer to the rather magical theories of the brilliant
Cambridge philosopher, Rupert Sheldrake. For some reason, however, the name often slips his memory. He fi-

nally solved the problem by associating "Sheldrake" with the name of a magician hero, "Mandrake," whose illustrated comic book stories had entertained him as a schoolboy when he should have been attending to his teachers.

◆ **Overcoming the Elusive Tip-of-the-Tongue Memory.** If someone's name is on the tip of your tongue, don't fight it. If you have the time, the best thing you can do is turn your attention to something else, and often the name will "pop up" in your mind after a while. This happens because several strong memories are competing with each other and blocking the recall of the information that you want. When you direct your attention to something else, all those memories weaken, but the incorrect memories weaken more.

Remembering to Take Your Medicine

Not taking medicine at the proper times or forgetting to take it at all is a major problem for doctors and patients. Remembering to take your medication, particularly if it is going to be a medication that you take long-term, is related to developing a habit. And habits are related to memory. We're willing to bet that when you first learned to drive you often didn't remember to take your car keys with you every time you left the house. Or maybe you forgot, left them in the ignition, and locked the car. Now you rarely if ever forget to take your keys with you. Why? Because it's become a habit. But that's only because you *learned* to carry those keys with you and now you automatically remember. Ditto for taking daily medicines which you can convert into a habit:

◆ **Strategically Place or Divide Your Containers.** If you take your medicine in the morning, keep the bottle beside your coffee cup. If you take it in the evening, place the container next to your toothbrush. If you take it both morning and evening, divide it into two bottles. Some people use a container that has seven compartments in it, one for each day of the week. That way, if you are not sure whether you took your pill earlier or not, you can check whether today's slot is empty.

◆ **Create Helpful Imagery.** Use some of the imagery techniques above to help you remember. Imagine your morning medication as a huge pill rising out of the cereal box or your coffee cup. Imagine your evening medication dancing on the bed. If you have to take medicine every so many hours, draw a clock face substituting the drawing of a pill at the times when you have to take the medicine and then keep the picture in a prominent place.

◆ **Use "Yellow Stickies."** We remember a high school English teacher who, when she had something out of the ordinary she had to remember, used a safety pin to attach a note to her dress. Sometimes when she had to remember a succession of things, or to take a temporary medicine several times during the day, she wore a chain of notes, which she removed, one at a time, as each task was accomplished or each pill taken. If you have someplace that you look at regularly during the day, you might put a "chain" of Post-it notes in that location, removing them from a left-handed position to a right-handed one each time you take a pill.

Bank Those Memories

In our busy lives as we go through one event after another, we simply cannot keep track of all the things we wanted to remember about that special day or that spectacular trip. We forget even some of our dearest experiences, and sadly this can happen at any age, even if our memories are otherwise pretty good and we have only minor signs of AAMI. To hold onto these memories, you have to do a little work:

◆ **Keep a Journal; Collect Small Mementos.** We suggest you establish a bank or deposit box of memories, but the contents will be different from your bank account or safety deposit box. One of the keys to the box might be a journal. Help preserve your memories with a daily journal, or if that is too much for you, then keep a journal of only special times, important events, your travels and journeys. One friend we know keeps a journal of her dreams, and sometimes rereading that journal reminds her of events that occurred or things she was working on in her personal life at the time. Sometimes she's simply astonished all over again at certain dreams and aware that she would have lost them without the journal. That same friend, a travel writer, keeps small mementos or tokens of her trips. They are another key to her memory bank. She need only look at those unusual rocks from Iceland to remember the day she bought them, the people she met, that part of the island, or, if she chooses, the whole trip around Iceland's Ring Road, which eventually led her to the stand where children were selling the rocks they had gathered.

◆ **Save Photos or Postcards.** If photos or videos are your thing, shoot scenes from your trip. If you don't want to carry a camera or other equipment, buy postcards, picture books, and/or tapes of local music. Make notes on the postcards for yourself, even mail them to yourself if you like. That way you'll also have a stamp of the country to compare to other countries.

◆ **Keep Contents of Your Memory Bank Visible.**

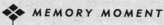

❖ MEMORY MOMENT _____

"*Some memories are realities, and are better than anything that can ever happen to one again.*"

—Willa Cather.

Don't store those souvenirs away. Frame the postcards or keep one on a tiny easel and change the postcards/photos frequently. Keep items around the house that remind you of wonderful experiences or exciting adventures such as that trip to Amsterdam. The wooden shoe sitting in front of a stack of books reminds you of the trip to Amsterdam, and that memory spirals into memories of other experiences in Holland. If you got your photo album out, you'd recover even more of those Dutch memories. Why not start putting memories in your memory bank today? The richness of your endeavor will pay off in the future.

Don't Forget the Internet

If you have a computer, you already have a valuable resource for improving your memory. There are sites where you can find free games. Your only cost will be the time and effort to download them. Some sites allow you to have a free preview of software memory games which, if you like a game, you can buy. Type in the address *http://www.search.com/?ctb.search*. Under the heading "computing," click the title "games download," and you will get a chance to type in what you are looking for. When we typed in "memory," we found 28 games, some for the Mac and some for the PC.

Another good site is *http://www.gamecenter.com/?st.gc.ss.pill.gc*, which specializes in all sorts of good games. Our search for memory games from this site revealed 30 references to memory games, many different from the site listed above.

Moraff's Memory-Jiggler is a unique combination of memory and jigsaw puzzles. Pieces flip over, but only stay faceup when they are in the right place. You can exchange any two pieces on the screen to get them in their right places. Discover this and other MoraffWare games at *http://www.winsite.com/info/pc/win3/games/ jiggler4.zip/SDN.ID* [no period].

It is never too late to take control of your ability to stimulate your mind and your life. Keep your neurons growing. Think of it as building brain branches, and strengthening and toning those neurons and their axons and dendrites. You can't do it all at once, but with steady practice and repetition, you will soon see the progress of your efforts. One thing is certain: at any age, you can have a better memory tomorrow than you have today.

Answers

Scrambled words: brain, synapse, memory, forgetting

The river puzzles:

1 The boy fills the four-cup can first and pours it into the three-cup can. He now has one cup left in the four-cup can.
2 The boy fills the eight-cup can and, from it, he fills the five-cup can. He empties the five-cup can, leaving him with three cups in the eight-cup can. He pours those into the now-empty five-cup can and fills up the eight-cup can, giving him a total of 11 cups.

3 The boy fills the four-cup can three times and empties it into the nine-cup can each time. The third time he goes to empty the four-cup can, the larger can will only hold one additional cup, leaving him three cups in the four-cup can.

How to shorten the line: Draw a three-inch line above it. Obviously, the lower line will be shorter! (Sorry!)

6

❖

Protect Your Health

Protect your health

◆

Watch your alcohol intake

◆

Say good-bye to cigarettes

◆

Avoid exposure to toxic materials

◆

Strengthen your immune system

◆

Use antioxidants

◆

Watch your weight and your food consumption

◆

Know your medications

◆

Do mental exercises

◆

Music and memory

◆

Principles for more effective memory

❖

Through the many studies reported in this book, you've learned that age-related memory loss is not inevitable, but is at least partially linked to factors that are under your control. This chapter will introduce you to additional ways to save your memory.

Early action will help prevent normal memory failure before it even starts, while following the Memory Cure, especially taking PS and exercising your memory regularly in middle age, may assure you a strong memory throughout your life—you can have a memory that largely or entirely escapes the effects of aging. The older we get, the greater the risk for disease, but, as a rule, that risk, especially for chronic disease, is greatly increased by an unhealthy lifestyle. Substantial research steadily accumulates to support the relationship between diet and good health.

Much of the variability found in the cognition of older individuals is a consequence of health-related factors. Some longitudinal studies show that many older people are able to retain cognitive performance that is not much lower than the standards of younger adults. The term "successful aging" has been introduced to take this into account. In successful aging, extrinsic factors often play an important role, and some experts think cognitive changes might be better explained not in terms of aging but rather in terms of such factors as lifestyle, habits, diet, and other psychosocial factors. While we do not fully agree with all of these views, we certainly do agree that these factors play an important role in age-related cognitive decline.

A study conducted at the Charles R. Drew University of Medicine and Science in Los Angeles on a sample of 1,250 African-American elderly individuals showed that more than 48.3 percent of the sample reported poor memory and forgetfulness as either a very serious or somewhat serious problem. Further examination of the data showed that complaints of memory problems were more likely to occur in those who had a hearing problem, reported a higher number of stressful life events, experienced a higher level of depression, and who suffered from poorer health in general.[109]

It is never too late to start protecting your health, plus there are some very specific things that you can do along the way to preserve and protect your memory whatever your age:

- ◆ Monitor your alcohol intake carefully.
- ◆ Don't smoke, or give it up if you already are a smoker.
- ◆ Strengthen your immune system.
- ◆ Add antioxidants to your diet so they can scavenge for free radicals.
- ◆ Watch your weight and your food consumption.
- ◆ Be sure you eat enough food of sufficient variety to provide ample amounts of nutrients important for mental functioning and to reinforce neurotransmitter production.
- ◆ Consider eating less, but avoid drastic dieting.
- ◆ Learn the side effects of any medication you have to take, and what you can do to balance any deficiencies it may cause.
- ◆ Never stop learning, thereby keeping your brain cells busy building dendritic spines.
- ◆ Make music an important part of your life.

Let's take a more detailed look at what we mean by each of these things.

Protect Your Health

When the newsletter *Bottom Line Personal* interviewed three of the country's leading doctors about the
health issues they personally face in their forties, fifties,
and sixties, all agreed that the key to good health—and
that also means brain longevity—is diet and exercise. It
is vitally important to adopt a lifestyle that involves the
appropriate amounts and types of foods, exercise a minimum of three times a week, and develop a repertoire of
techniques, hobbies, etc., that allows you to reduce stress
when needed. Exercise itself is also a good stress reducer,
and it helps you burn calories and keep weight down. It
also helps strengthen the heart, improve blood flow, and
reduce cholesterol levels.[110]

Excess weight plays a part in a number of health problems: high blood pressure (hypertension), diabetes, and
heart disease—and some even think it plays a role in the
development of cancer. Hypertension, diabetes, and heart
disease can all be damaging to all cognitive function including memory. Also, excess fat increases free radical
production, which is harmful to neurons.

Dr. Timothy McCall, an internist in the Boston area
who is in his forties, said that "life in your forties is
about balance and setting one's sights on the long
term."[111] He calls it the "Decade of Prevention," because
much of what we do at that time creates habits that will
endure for the rest of our lives. Dr. Bernadine Healy, in
her fifties, is Dean of the College of Medicine and Public
Health at the Ohio State University in Columbus and former Director of the National Institutes of Health. She
thinks the fifties are a prime time to change your pattern
of eating, especially since it is a time when most of us
are increasingly vulnerable to diseases that affect longev-

ity, and eating too much or the wrong kind of food heightens the chances that we will be affected by them.

Dr. William Castelli, a respected expert on epidemiology and prevention of heart disease, now in his sixties, states that by the time we reach this decade, our levels of cholesterol, blood pressure, and blood sugar will play a major role "in whether or not we sail through the rest of our lives without getting into trouble with illness."[112]

All three doctors stated that a healthy diet is one rich in fruits and vegetables (five servings a day) and whole grains, and low in saturated fats (to reduce the risk of heart disease and cancer). Most have cut down on red meat and have added more fish to their diet to obtain the extra heart protection offered by the omega-3 fatty acids. They exercise from 30 to 45 minutes at least four times a week. (Diet and exercise topics are covered in each issue of Brenda Adderly's newsletter, *Health Watch*.)

Watch Your Alcohol Intake

Your memory is intricately bound up with your physical state of being and is, therefore, vulnerable to any kind of physical abuse, especially that of chemical or substance abuse. Excessive alcohol intake is the second leading cause of preventable death in the United States and a common cause of mental decline in old age.[113]

There is a considerable body of evidence that moderate alcohol intake offers protection against heart disease by improving the HDL ("good" cholesterol) to LDL ("bad" cholesterol) ratio. However, heavy drinking contributes to liver disease, a variety of cancers, a weakening of the heart muscle, high blood pressure, strokes, and depression. Dr. Charles H. Hennekens, associate editor of *Health News* and a professor at Harvard Medical School, definitely states the obvious when he says that the health benefits of an alcoholic drink a day are "substantially smaller than those offered by exercise and eating right."[114] While alcohol in small quantities dilates the blood vessels of the brain, higher quantities induce their constriction, reducing cerebral blood flow, and—although this has not been proven—may reduce cognitive function and memory.[115]

The neuropsychological deficits observed in alcoholics appear to be larger in older alcoholics, leading some researchers to suspect that alcohol promotes *premature* aging of the brain, although the issue has yet to be studied in any great detail.[116] In one of the early studies on the effect of alcohol ingestion on memory, the negative effect of alcohol on recognition speed and rate of forgetting was demonstrated with a technique that required subjects to give an old or new response to each of 200 items presented sequentially on a computer screen (95 items appeared twice).[117] Since then, many studies have also demonstrated that alcohol interferes with short-term memory. If you impair your ability to retain new information, you have no chance to transform it into long-term memory.

As we grow older, most of us have less tolerance for alcohol; it takes fewer drinks to reach a state of inebriation and memory impairment. The problem for youthful alcohol drinkers is just the opposite. Alcohol doesn't make young brains as sleepy as it does adults' brains. Young rats injected with alcohol took longer to fall asleep and slept less than half the length of time of adult rats so injected. Alcohol inhibits the excitatory amino acid receptors of the hippocampus, which play an important role in the acquisition and storage of new information.[118] And it does so to a greater degree in immature animals as opposed to more mature animals. Translated to humans, this could mean that, although the youthful brain is capable of staying awake through long bouts of drinking, at the same time, any excess alcohol consumption, say two stiff drinks on top of each other, can inhibit learning and memory. The youthful brain is sustaining far more damage to memory and learning systems than an adult brain receiving an equivalent amount of alcohol.[119]

Frequently, we hear more about the problems of prenatal exposure to alcohol. It has been associated with birth defects running the gamut from severe physical problems to mental retardation to much more subtle compromises of cognitive functioning. Evidence from studies with laboratory animals shows that the hippocampus is damaged both structurally and neurochemically after in-utero exposure to alcohol.[120]

What this means is that, while alcohol in moderation—say one drink with dinner and one late in the evening—is probably more beneficial than not, several drinks before dinner followed by a bottle of wine will decrease your ability to concentrate, learn, and remember.

Say Good-bye to Cigarettes

Cigarette smoking lowers the amount of oxygen that gets to the brain. While dilation of the blood vessels in the brain occurs immediately after cigarette smoking, chronic smoking slows the overall reduction in cerebral blood flow. It also causes vasoconstriction of the blood vessels in other areas of the body, and infuses the red blood cells with carbon monoxide, greatly reducing their oxygen-carrying capacity. In a sense, this constitutes a slow suffocation of the cells in the body and is far more pernicious than any possible benefit that might accrue from nicotine, which, as some research has shown, in small quantities may temporarily "wake up" certain aspects of memory.

Smoking also greatly increases the number of free radicals in the blood. Eventually it affects the lungs and hinders breathing, which depletes energy and strength.

Although the effects of cigarette smoking on a variety of diseases, including cancer and cardiovascular illness and emphysema, have been well publicized, the effect of smoking on nutrients in the body are less widely known. Consider the destructive effects of cadmium, a toxic trace element as deadly as mercury and lead, and one of the components of tobacco. One pack of cigarettes yields 10 times the amount of cadmium the body is capable of assimilating, thus weaking the immune system.[121] Cadmium gets into tobacco in several ways, most commonly from growing tobacco in cadmium-polluted soil. In *Toxic Metal Syndrome,* Drs. Morton D. Walker and Richard H. Casdorph explain that cadmium is sprayed on tobacco as a fungicide. Even if you don't smoke, environmental exposure to tobacco smoke raises your blood concentration of cadmium.[122] Israeli investigators found that the blood levels of cadmium in nonsmokers exposed to cigarette smoke was very close to the average found in smokers.[123]

Cadmium decreases the availability of selenium and inhibits the metabolism of zinc. Not only does smoking lower the level of Vitamin C and beta-carotene in the blood and reduce levels of Vitamin E and several B-complex vitamins in body tissues, but for unknown reasons smokers also are less likely to consume fruits and vegetables, particularly those high in Vitamin C and carotenes.[124]

Studies have shown that smokers have more difficulty remembering people's faces and names than nonsmokers. To further complicate the issue, a five-year study of 1,007 young adults in the Detroit area found that people diagnosed with major depression are three times more likely to become smokers, and daily smokers are nearly twice as likely to be diagnosed with depression.[125] Depression, as we have seen, adversely affects memory.

The effects of smoking in combination with chronic alcoholism compound the problems of cognitive impairment. A French study and a study conducted at the University of Michigan both determined that there is a definitive correlation between the severity of alcohol dependence and the severity of nicotine dependence.[126] Alcoholics smoked more heavily and experienced higher rates of discomfort and nicotine withdrawal symptoms upon smoking cessation.[127] Although only about 10 percent of the population are heavy smokers, among alcoholics, 70 to 90 percent are heavy smokers.

The fact of the matter is that, for any number of reasons, including its adverse effect on your memory, you should not smoke. But then, no doubt, you already knew that smoking is bad for your health!

Avoid Exposure to Toxic Materials

It is well known that the effects of lead poisoning on the central nervous system include the lowering of I.Q., and the impairment of memory, reaction time, and the ability to concentrate. What is not so well known is how pervasive the problem is. In the United States alone, from 3 to 4 million children have lead poisoning. It affects one in every six children under the age of six.[128] You can minimize your exposure to lead paint by making sure that, if you intend to move into an older house or office building that appears to have old or flaking paint, you make sure to have it analyzed for lead content. The chances are there will be no problem. But it's better to be safe.

Another potential memory hazard is exposure to solvents as used in paints, paint thinners, and some industrial cleaning products. Extended use of such products harms memory. Thirty-eight journeymen painters and 36 nonexposed control participants were recruited from the Pittsburgh area. The painters were tested shortly after having worked with solvent-based paints, or after an interval when they had not painted for at least five days. Overall results showed that all the painters had significantly lower scores than controls on the majority of cognitive tests used in the study, and that painters tested soon after painting performed the worst on tests of learning and memory.[129]

Strengthen Your Immune System

Anything you can do to boost your immune system will help you avoid illnesses that require memory-robbing medication or that can result in reduced memory themselves. Low immunity leaves you more susceptible to bacterial and viral infections. In American hospitals, where many patients are taking drugs that undermine the immune system, roughly 2 million patients a year become ill with just such infections, adding to their health costs and further contributing to the general weakening of their immune systems.[130]

Some science writers have a tendency to talk about the

immune system as if it were the body's "department of defense." In fact, the immune system lacks a "headquarters" or central organ. Rather, it is a complete system comprised of a variety of organs in the body, including the skin, mucous membranes, tonsils and adenoids, thymus, spleen, lymph nodes, appendix, bone marrow, and certain areas of the small intestine. Within the blood are a variety of white blood cells that have differing functions and form a network of cells to fight various invaders, such as allergens, viruses, bacteria, and "foreign" cells like cancer. Among the many white blood cells are the T (for thymus-derived) lymphocytes, B cells (B for bone marrow), phagocytes (scavengers that devour debris in tissue and the bloodstream), killer T-cells, and suppressor cells.

It is known that immune cells and nerve cells interact. Receptors for chemicals released during stress (epinephrine and norepinephrine) have been observed on the surface of lymphocytes that are found near nerve terminals in the lymph nodes and spleen. This suggests that "what goes on in the brain can interact with the immune system to suppress or, conversely, enhance its action."[131] Clearly, then, weakening your immune system is going to harm your memory, perhaps directly by making you more susceptible to AD and other brain-debilitating diseases (although this has not been proven), and certainly by making you more vulnerable to many diseases that impair memory.

PS AIDS THE IMMUNE SYSTEM

Experiments with laboratory animals show that there are "recognition sites" in the immune cells of rats and PS reaches and activates those cells.[132] Some researchers have proposed applying the term "autocoid" to the ability of PS to activate defense reactions in the immune system.[133]

What, then, is the best way to boost your immune system? We know you've heard it before, but we can't say it often enough: In addition to taking your daily dose of PS, eat a varied, balanced diet of vegetables, fruits, grains, low-fat dairy products, and some fish and meat.

Use Antioxidants

Antioxidants are crucial to your efforts to protect your brain cells. We discuss antioxidants in detail in Chapter 7, but some further research studies are worth noting. For instance, a 22-year study, published in 1997, demonstrated that high levels of antioxidants in the blood of people aged 65 and older are associated with better memory performance.

The plasma levels of alpha-tocopherol (Vitamin E), ascorbic acid (Vitamin C), and beta-carotene (converted to Vitamin A in the body) of 444 people—312 men and 132 women—aged 65 to 94 years in Basel, Switzerland, were first measured in 1971 and then again in 1993. The group was selected from a random sample of the population of Basel, a town that is considered representative of the older urban population in Switzerland. Men and women who had a high intake of food rich in ascorbic acid and beta-carotene, or who had taken supplements, scored significantly higher on tests of semantic memory than did similar adults who had low vitamin levels.[134]

Watch Your Weight and Your Food Consumption

Less fat, more carbohydrates. For some time now, that's been the message of the U.S. Department of Agriculture's dietary guidelines designed to help prevent chronic diseases. Continuing research suggests that the *type* of fat is more important than the amount of fat. Unfortunately, Americans have apparently decided the "less fat" advice means that we can eat a lot more, according to registered dietitian Julia Walsh. Consequently, the intake of calories for Americans has shot up more than 200 calories a day.[135] So, alas, not only do we have to watch the fats, but we also have to remain aware of calorie consumption. Saturated fats are chains "saturated" with hydrogen molecules. Consequently, they are less able to be oxidized (i.e., burned) for energy. Instead, they are more likely to deposit in our arteries—and, not infrequently, on our hips! They're abundant in meat, poultry, butter, cheese, milk, and cream, as well as coconut, palm, and palm kernel oils. Although the current intake of saturated fats seems to run around 12 percent of total calories daily, Walsh recommends it should be no more than 8 percent of calories. This means only small amounts of these items in your diet.

Monounsaturated fats have one free spot to which oxygen molecules can attach. Some of the best sources are olive oil and canola oil, peanut oil and peanuts. Walsh recommends that monounsaturated fats make up 12 to 20 percent of total calories.

Polyunsaturated fats have two or more free spots available for oxygen to grab onto. The two main families of poly fats are the omega-6 and omega-3 fats. The omega fats are called "essential" fatty acids because the body can't make them, yet must manufacture all the other fats it needs from them. The primary omega-6 fat is linoleic acid. Omega-6 fats lower blood levels of cholesterol, and good sources are soybeans, and corn, sunflower, and safflower oils. The omega-3 fatty acids are alpha linolenic

acid or LNA (contained in plants), eicosaphntaenoic acid
(EPA), and decoahexaenoic acid (DHA). Linolenic acid
is found in fish and fish oils, walnuts, walnut oil, and
flaxseed oil. In general, fish that live in deep, cold water
have higher levels of omega-3's. This means mackerel,
lake trout, chinook and Atlantic salmon, lake whitefish,
and tuna. Omega-3's reduce blood clotting, prevent abnormal heart rhythms, improve immune function, and
promote eye and brain development.

Dr. Artemis P. Simopoulos, president of the Center
for Genetics, Nutrition and Health in Washington, D.C.,
advises that, contrary to earlier research that indicated
only one meal of fish per week would confer significant
protection against heart attack, more recent studies show
it is better to eat fish two or three times a week. Eating
fish more frequently than that does not seem to provide
any additional protection, says Dr. Simopoulos, who also
advises that you can get omega-3 acids in capsules sold
at health-food stores. The important thing to watch with
supplements is how much EPA and DHA they contain.
You should be getting about 1 gram of both each day. If
you take capsules, take them with meals to ensure that
the fish oil is properly absorbed. The minimum amount
of LNA obtained from plant sources should be 6 grams
per day.[136] However, since there is no easy way to determine how much you are getting, taking the supplement
is probably a good idea.

Trans unsaturated fatty acids ("trans fats") have been
very much in the news. These sinister fats form when
vegetable oils have hydrogen chemically added to make
them solid at room temperature and able to withstand
frying temperatures. They are found in stick margarines,
shortening, pastries, packaged cookies, crackers, french
fries, and other deep-fried foods. They have been linked

to breast cancer and an increased risk of coronary heart disease. Avoid these as much as possible. Although manufacturers don't have to include information on trans fats in their "nutrition facts" boxes, you can satisfy yourself by looking for the dead-giveaway word "hydrogenated."

AVOID POOR NUTRITION

Studies of learning and memory ability during periods of being well-nourished or undernourished have been done, largely with rats, but they have important implications for older adults who may not be eating well or who are eating a limited range of foods.

Rats that were either fed well or kept undernourished during their suckling and early post-weaning periods (birth to 45 days) were exposed to shape stimuli (triangles and circles) beginning on the twenty-fifth day and extending to the forty-fifth day. Beginning on day 132, the ability to discriminate the shapes was tested. Improved learning performance occurred only in the well-nourished rats, while undernutrition interfered with the "incidental learning" (learning about features of the environment that are not, at the time, biologically relevant) in undernourished rats.[137]

In Japan, the concentration of tryptophan (the "relaxing" neurotransmitter) in the brain decreased and the total number of correct responses in a brightness discrimination test (akin to memory) increased for rats fed a diet enriched with certain amino acids (methionine and threonine) compared to rats on a low soy protein diet.[138]

A lifelong diet low in fat prevents so many health problems that occur with aging—and that can affect memory—that we must continually recommend it. It is important to eat fresh fruits and vegetables, whole grain cereals/breads, and low-fat dairy foods daily. Small, frequent meals (snacks of the right kind) may be easier to eat or prepare than larger ones, and studies show that this kind of eating—sometimes called "grazing"—is actually better for the body in terms of blood sugar (glucose) and energy levels.

If you have access to the worldwide web on the Internet, you can get an evaluation of your intake of nutrients—based on daily allowance data from the U.S. Department of Agriculture—from the Illinois Council on Food and Agricultural Research at the University of Illinois at Urbana-Champaign (*www.spectre.ag.uiuc.edu/ ~food-lab/nat/*). The program will also recommend alternatives for more nutritious dining. (You can also look to Brenda Adderly's *Health Watch* newsletter, which features a new, delicious, low-fat meal each month.)

DON'T DIET DRASTICALLY . . .

A study that took a first look at the effect of dieting on the cognitive performance of 70 women showed that the 15 women who were dieting displayed impaired performance on a vigilance task and tended to show poorer immediate memory and longer reaction times. They did show a better performance on an undemanding finger-tapping task than women who were normally highly restrained eaters and women who were not dieting. Highly restrained eaters who were not dieting at the time of testing typically performed at an intermediate level on the cognitive tests. The authors suggest that poorer cognitive functioning during dieting could arise as a direct consequence of the effects of food restriction on energy metabolism (dieters were eating at about 70 percent of maintenance energy requirements) or as a result of anxiety resulting from the stressful effects of imposing and maintaining dietary restraint.[139]

We're not giving you permission here to gobble up everything in sight. Rather we're suggesting that you eat in such a way as to control your weight in the first place, so you don't have to experience the memory deficits incurred during dieting. Try eating six or eight small meals spaced out during the day to keep refueling your brain and keep your blood sugar level on an even keel. Remember, the brain uses about 20 percent of the body's blood sugar when it's resting, and even higher levels while concentrating or performing other mental tasks during the day. As you saw earlier, depending on its severity, hypoglycemia or low blood sugar can create a number of mental symptoms that interfere with cognitive functioning.

. . . BUT DO CONSIDER CALORIE RESTRICTION

Some research in the 1970s showed that calorie-restricted mice lived 30 percent to 50 percent longer than mice allowed to eat as much as they wanted. Caloric restriction also prevented the decline of dopamine receptors in their brain cells. A more recent study showed that for mice, a caloric reduction that occurred at midlife increased longevity, preserved strength and coordination, and prolonged some types of cognitive maze functioning.[140]

We're not talking, however, about the intensive reduction in calories that most diets require, but rather the kind of calorie restriction adopted by the eight-person team that lived for two years (from September 26, 1991, to September 26, 1993) in Biosphere 2, a self-contained habitat in the Arizona desert. Because the group could only eat what they grew within the dome, they typically lived on a 2,200 calorie diet (as Dr. Roy L. Walford, the resident physician for the Biosphere group, continues to do) compared to the 2,500 to 3,300 calories they were used to eating. Blood pressure, blood sugar, insulin, and cholesterol levels all fell. Dr. Walford, a longtime guru for calorie restriction, believes that our bodies evolved to survive food shortages by shifting available energy from growth and reproduction to repair.[141]

Dr. Walford advises that, if you want to try calorie restriction, the trick is to eat plenty of fruits, vegetables, beans, grains, and tofu. Don't make meats and dairy products the primary focus of your meals. Also, eat more "nutrient-dense" foods such as wheat germ, oat bran, brewer's yeast, and seaweed, all of which you can add to soups, salads, cereals, and casseroles. Cut back on the consumption of sugar, alcohol, butter, and other fats. Unlike the group of women we mentioned above in the Don't Diet section, you should not attempt to reduce calorie intake by more than 30 percent.

Know Your Medications

Some medications, both prescription and over-the-counter, can make you feel unfocused, thus slowing down your recall and making it hard to direct your attention and concentrate. Many drugs widely used as sleep aids and antidepressants can have profound negative effects on the brain.[142]

As people grow older, they tend to take more medications. While a single medication may not cause cognitive impairment—although some will—combinations of drugs can often cause cognitive problems that mimic more serious diseases. While drug-related cognitive deterioration occurs in only 5 percent of the population, when you consider that the middle-aged and elderly population numbers in the tens of millions, this is nevertheless a problem that affects many people.[143] Therefore, if you develop a memory problem within a couple of days after starting to take a medication, promptly check with your doctor. Also check if you have been taking a medication for some time and suddenly develop cognitive difficulties. Possibly your brain may have become more sensitive to the medication with aging or long-term ingestion, or the addition of a new medication to your prescription regime may be the culprit.

One study showed that among 300 elderly patients evaluated for cognitive impairment, 35 had adverse drug reactions that were producing the symptoms. The relative odds of an adverse reaction associated with cognitive impairment increase as the number of prescription drugs increases.[144] Drugs for sleep or anxiety, such as the benzodiazepines, have a particularly high risk of cognitive impairment (see Chapter 7).

Other drugs associated with a risk of cognitive impairment include certain antihypertensive agents, sedating antipsychotic drugs, opioids, digitalis, anti-Parkinsonian drugs, antidepressants, and corticosteroids.[145] Medicine should always be considered a possible cause when there is a memory problem or confusion, but *do not stop taking a prescription medication unless your doctor advises it.*[146]

If you develop any memory or reasoning problems, make a list of all the medications you take, plus your alcohol consumption (if any), and ask your doctor if your particular combination of drugs can impair cognition. If you are unable to discontinue the use of some medications, ask your doctor to consider adjustments in dosage amounts or the substitution of another drug that may produce less of a problem.

(More scary, and a good reason to maintain your health, is the statistic that in 1994 between 76,000 and

137,000 people died from adverse drug reactions, ranking it somewhere between the fourth and sixth leading cause of death in the United States. Taking the midpoint of 106,000 drug-induced deaths means that three out of every thousand patients had a fatal reaction.[147])

If you must take medication, it becomes crucial that you know about the potential problems and the risk-benefit ratio of any medications prescribed for you. Drugs that cause the most serious medical problems in hospitalized patients are painkillers, antibiotics and antiviral drugs, and cardiovascular and anticoagulant drugs.

Do Mental Exercises

Whatever your age, ongoing mental stimulation will keep your brain building new spines on the dendrites of your brain cells. Your "communication tree" will keep branching. We've covered this before, so there's no point in repeating it here except to reemphasize that nothing (except taking PS) will do more to delay the loss of memory than constant mental exercise.

Importantly, this applies at any age. And it's a question of challenge. So . . .

- ◆ Limit your television viewing to shows that teach you something. Avoid what someone has called "television pap."
- ◆ Choose novels that are not "page-turners" but rather thought-provokers.
- ◆ Strive for a job where originality rather than "doing it our way" is rewarded.
- ◆ Don't retire! By all means quit your job if you want, but make certain you have a new "career" with enough momentum to it to keep you mentally

busy and on your toes. (You don't have to make money; but you should make *something!*)

Music and Memory

In monasteries in Brittany, cows serenaded with music give more milk. In northern Japan music increases by a factor of 10 the density of a yeast used to make sake, the traditional Japanese rice wine. It is what Don Campbell, musician, educator, and author of a book by the same name, calls "The Mozart Effect."

Campbell's book contains many heartwarming anecdotes of healing with music. Because the studies are difficult to re-create in the laboratory, many researchers question the validity of the Mozart effect. One of the first studies to attempt to re-create the Mozart effect in the laboratory was conducted in the mid-1990s in the Center for Neurobiology of Learning and Memory at the University of California, Irvine. There researchers conducted a first study and then replicated their results with a second study, showing that listening to a Mozart piano sonata produced significant short-term enhancement of spatial-temporal reasoning in college students.[148] Later studies employing electroencephalogram (EEG) recordings showed that the music produced activity in the right frontal and left temporo-parietal lobes.[149]

Some of the same Irvine researchers later were able to show that private piano lessons improved the spatial-temporal reasoning and spatial recognition of preschool children significantly more than did private computer lessons, suggesting that music training might produce long-term modifications in underlying neural circuitry in regions not primarily concerned with music.[150]

Sixteen female and 16 male undergraduates showed a

small but significant improvement in spatial learning tests following the presentation of Mozart's Sonata for Two Pianos in D Major.[151]

While memory was not measured per se in these various tests, the improvements shown were such that we can reasonably postulate that a memory improvement would have shown up had the researchers been looking for it.

In his book, Campbell reported extensively on the work, during the last half-century, of Dr. Alfred Tomatis. A French physician, Dr. Tomatis has developed a unique program for healing all kinds of physical and psychological problems with music. Dr. Tomatis believes that the most stimulating and changing aspects of sound are in the high-frequency range and that these sounds help activate our brains and increase attentiveness.[152]

Contradictory evidence began to accumulate in the mid- to late 1990s regarding the effect of music on learning, especially spatial learning or reasoning, and on memory. None of the studies made any attempt to reproduce the kind of environments discussed in Campbell's book. Some research suggested that a 10-minute or more exposure to classical music can significantly influence the performance on a spatial task,[153] although in many studies the effect has not been dramatic, and inconsistent results may be due to a sensitivity in individuals or the fact that music, being so widely variant, could be expected to have many different effects.

For example, when two cognitive tests were conducted with college students, one in silence and the other with background music, more questions were completed and more answers were correct with the musical background.[154] On the other hand, one unusual study investigated the features of instrumental background music that would interfere with serial recall for visually presented

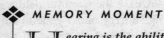

❖ MEMORY MOMENT _____

Hearing is the ability to receive auditory information through our senses, listening is the ability "to filter, selectively focus on, remember, and respond to sound."[155]

—Don Campbell.

items. Twenty-four students were presented sequences of nine digits and required to recall the digits in order of presentation. Background instrumental music played forward caused significantly more disruption than did either silence or background instrumental music played backward.[156]

Similarly, we know that "easy-listening" music can slow down heartbeat, pulse rate, and blood pressure. But music with a strong beat has just the opposite effect. If you've ever experienced a sense of joy or a "natural high" from listening to music, then you've already learned that music can increase the release of endorphins (the body's natural painkillers) from the pituitary.

Listening to music decreases the agitation and increases the focus and concentration of people with Alzheimer's disease (AD). One study found that people with AD could recall the words to songs better than spoken words or information, enabling family members or caregivers to engage in vocal communication.[157]

Music can boost the immune function. Singing, chanting, and some other forms of vocalization exercises can oxygenate the cells, and raise the level of interleukins in the blood, and has been shown to increase lymphatic circulation as high as three times the normal rate. It has also been found to decrease levels of cortisol, break down cancer cells, and to relieve severe depression.[158]

Music can reduce pain and decrease the need for analgesia. When patients undergoing surgery under general anesthesia wore headphones and listened to music in the post-anesthesia care unit (PACU), there was no difference in pain level, morphine requirement, respiration, or length of stay in PACU between the "listening" group and two groups that did not hear music, yet the music group was able to wait significantly longer before requiring analgesia. Members of this group also perceived their PACU experience as significantly more pleasant than the patients in the other two groups as recalled on both day one and after one month.[159]

The method of using Baroque music to assist in learning developed by Bulgarian psychologist Georgi Lozanov, and popularized in the international best-seller *Superlearning 2000* by Sheila Ostrander and Lynn Shroeder, appears to bring learners into a state of alert relaxation. Schools and individuals who have used it find it particularly effective for memorizing spelling words and poetry, and for learning foreign languages.[160]

So, while you're adding supplements, exercise, and the right food to your lifestyle, don't forget to add a little Mozart. It should help your memory. But if you find it doesn't, well, there's an easy solution: turn it off!

 MEMORY MOMENT

> " In memory everything seems to happen to music."
>
> —Tom Wingfield,
> in Tennessee Williams's
> *The Glass Menagerie.*

Principles for More Effective Memory

Here are some general guidelines to help you make the most of your memory:

1 Make a conscious effort to exercise your memory *every day,* even if it is only to practice memorizing a list. Decide what you want to remember and then pick a strategy from the Memory Maximizer techniques in Chapter 5 and practice it. In this way you will begin to recognize which techniques work best for you.

2 Most of us are better at problem-solving in the morning, so train your mind with word games and mind teasers before lunch. "Morning people" probably already know that they do their best learning in the morning. Their ability to retain learned material decreases as the day continues, while that of "evening people" may stay level or even improve as the day extends.[161]

3 Memorize important facts or concepts shortly before you go to sleep. Since 1924, studies have shown that information learned just before sleep is retained better, and these studies have been duplicated many times since.

4 Make use of spacing. If you must have marathon memory sessions, don't try to memorize all you need to know at one time. Break up your study periods into time spans of about 90 minutes, or whatever you have discovered is most comfortable for you. Then take a break before you go back to work. One psychology colleague told us of discovering for himself that he could most effectively study for his doctoral exams by working intensely for 90 min-

utes, then taking a 10-minute break to mow part of the lawn before returning to study another 90 minutes. It took the lawn longer to get mowed, but it increased the efficiency of his studying.

5 Practice, practice, practice; but don't overload your practice with too many techniques or for too long a time. Researchers have found that the most effective training programs for learning/retention have been those in which intensive (usually one-hour) training has focused on one particular technique or strategy at a time. Many of us have poor but ingrained methods of memorizing. Successful retraining takes time and effort. It also requires you to want to learn to memorize or remember better, and to develop the confidence that you can learn new techniques. Research shows that there are plenty of memory tricks out there waiting to be learned and utilized.

If you follow the precepts of this chapter from the very moment that you first observe the slightest memory decline—or, even better, before you notice any and only because you have reached your fiftieth birthday (perhaps the one event you *don't* want to remember!)—there is every reason to believe that, for decades to come, your memory will remain intact. In some ways, it may even improve.

7

❖

PS-Boosting Supplements

Always talk to your doctor first

◆

Supplements that boost the effectiveness of PS

◆

The need for nutritional supplements

◆

The memory minerals

◆

Is food medicine?

❖

For years, European doctors, health-food advocates, nutritionists, and other health-food workers have touted the brain-boosting qualities of a number of vitamins, antioxidants, herbs, and minerals. Unfortunately, there has been a great deal of wishful thinking—and also quite a bit of plain nonsense—written about these supplements. And quite a bit of that has found its way across the Atlantic. In this chapter, therefore, we shall provide you with the best information available about which nutritional supplements work, which may work but are unproven, and which don't. Then, in a later chapter, we shall discuss a number of prescription drugs, some avail-

able only outside the United States, said to help boost
memory and/or slow the rate of AAMI, and give you a
sense of how helpful, if at all, those may be.

For the sake of clarity, we've broken this chapter into
three parts:

◆ First, we'll cover those nutritional supplements
  that are said to directly improve memory. It's a list
  of only three, and our overall conclusion is that
  these supplements have only a marginal effect
  when used alone. They may boost the effectiveness
  of PS, however, when taken in conjunction with it.

◆ Second, we shall cover a list of vitamins, minerals,
  and other supplements that don't work directly on
  memory, but do strengthen aspects of our minds
  and bodies that are necessary to permit our memories to function at their optimum efficiency.

◆ Finally, we shall provide some important nutritional guidelines that will boost your overall
  health—and avoid unnecessary illness—and thus
  maximize your physical and mental energy and vitality. No doubt, such heightened "blooming good
  health" will be beneficial to your memory, if for
  no other reason than that it will give you the vigor
  to implement our other memory-boosting recommendations.

Always Talk to Your Doctor First

While the term "alternative medicine" is widely used
to describe a health-care approach that includes therapeutic use of nutritional supplements or "nutraceuti-
cals"—as well as a wide-ranging series of other therapies,
ranging from acupuncture to baby massage to the use of

magnets—we prefer the term "complementary medicine." That is because we feel strongly that natural healing methods, valuable though they are in themselves, are far more valuable when used, under the guidance of an open-minded physician in conjunction with carefully researched, laser-targeted, and often miraculously effective pharmaceutical drugs. For example, most of the medical profession now agrees with the once controversial views that a mixture of glucosamine and chondroitin sulfate can halt, reverse, or even cure osteoarthritis. In fact, Brenda Adderly has written books on these subjects. But we would never advocate using natural healing methods *instead* of using traditional medicine to cure the cause of the pain, ensure your baby is healthy, or operate on arthritic knees too deteriorated to respond to the supplements. Rather, we are convinced that our "complementary" recommendations work far more effectively when used in conjunction with the best of conventional medicine.

Therefore, before you use PS or any of the supplements discussed in this chapter, we strongly urge you to discuss them with your doctor so that together you can build a medical-nutritional regimen that is exactly tailored to your specific health needs.

Having said that, let us add that, while we feel confident that the supplements we present in this chapter are safe and without side effects (except as we shall mention), you should be aware that they may possibly interact with other medications you are taking. For instance, a potential problem with the use of both gingko and ginseng is that, since they are blood thinners, combining them with prescription anticoagulant drugs, even aspirin, could cause internal bleeding or might even possibly contribute to a stroke.[162]

Supplements That Boost the Effectiveness of PS

GINKGO BILOBA

Having first appeared about 200 million years ago *Ginkgo biloba,* a native of China, is the oldest surviving species of tree on earth. Now grown all over the world, ginkgo is the only thing that contains *ginkgolides,* unique substances that are known to have vasodilating (blood-vessel widening) properties. They also have potent antioxidant benefits that block free radical damage.

Ginkgo has been very widely researched, usually in the form of a standardized ginkgo extract known as EGb 761, which is a purified, complex mixture of chemicals obtained from ginkgo leaves and manufactured by Wilmar Schwabe GMBH of Karlsruhe, Germany. And EGb 761 has received the German government's approval for the treatment of Alzheimer's disease (AD). Here is what we know generally about ginkgo and its impact on memory:

- ◆ Ginkgo improves blood flow. Used as a standard treatment in Europe for people with blood circulation problems, ginkgo decreases "blood stickiness," and increases the elasticity of tiny blood vessels. Each of these functions improves blood flow in the brain, which is one reason that ginkgo is popularly touted to improve memory.
- ◆ Ginkgo blocks the shrinkage of the hippocampus. This part of the brain plays a critical role in memory. It may shrink due to stress, or as a normal condition of aging. In theory, ginkgo's ability to help reduce this shrinkage should improve memory or, at least, block its long-term decline.
- ◆ Ginkgo is an effective antioxidant. Animal studies

provide some support for the thesis that ginkgo is an unusually effective antioxidant. For example, it is effective in protecting animals' retinal tissue against damage by free radicals, which most other supplements can't do.[163] While this characteristic has nothing to do with memory, it provides a hint that ginkgo may be effective in preventing free radical damage in the brain—and, if this were so, ginkgo would help memory. Similarly, ginkgo has other health benefits, ranging from protecting rats' optic nerves from damage caused by diabetes,[164] to reducing the sleeping time of anesthetized mice.[165] Again, these studies obviously are far afield from memory, but they do support the widely held view that ginkgo is a valuable and potent antioxidant healer, and they therefore serve as the backdrop against which the surge of enthusiasm for ginkgo as a memory booster must be evaluated.

When it comes to studies conducted directly on the effectiveness of ginkgo for memory, there is a very large body of research that has some bearing. However, the results of the research are somewhat mixed.

In laboratory mice, the extract significantly improved short-term memory and membrane fluidity, but did not improve long-term memory.[166] Other European research has shown that EGb 761 protects neuronal cell membranes from free radical damage in aging mice, and so improves their cognitive functions and presumably memories. Recently Dr. Jerrold C. Winter of the State University of New York at Buffalo, determined that not only did EGb 761 improve the memory of rats, but it also significantly prolonged their life compared to rats not receiving ginkgo.[167]

To see whether ginkgo has the same memory-booster quality for humans, and to try to confirm the many and varied reports about ginkgo's putative efficacy, a team of American psychiatrists from several university medical schools, led by Pierre Le Bars, M.D., Ph.D., conducted a one-year, randomized, double-blind, placebo-controlled study of 309 patients with mild to severe dementia from AD and other causes. Published in the *Journal of the American Medical Association (JAMA),* this study caused a great flurry in the American press and among consumers, and boosted sales of ginkgo at least threefold. However, the furor was based on an exaggerated understanding of the findings of this study. In fact, of the 202 patients who completed the trial, there were only modest, although statistically significant, increases (or slow downs in the rate of deterioration) in cognitive performance including memory and recognizable improvement in social functioning, for those taking EGb 761.[168] (Social functioning is not the same as memory, of course, but it involves memory and therefore is seen by ginkgo advocates as demonstrating that ginkgo works.) However, the American medical and scientific community questioned part of the research methodology, and therefore expressed skepticism about the study's findings. Nevertheless, the researchers, more optimistic than others, concluded that, "EGb was safe and appears capable of stabilizing and, in a substantial number of cases, improving the cognitive performance and the social functioning of demented patients for 6 months to 1 year. Although modest, the changes induced by EGb were . . . of sufficient magnitude to be recognized by the care givers. . . ."[169]

Ginkgo, then, may offer some small benefit to patients suffering from AD. However, nothing in this study sug-

gests that ginkgo would be helpful for ordinary AAMI.
Moreover, since ginkgo seems to gain its main impact
from vasodilation, not from rebuilding or blocking the
degradation of any part of the brain's cellular structure,
there is not much reason to believe that it will act prophylactically to block the onset of AAMI, which is not, in
most cases, due to restricted blood circulation.

◆ In 1992, a group of German scientists, led by E.
   Grassel, studied the effects of ginkgo on the short-
   term memory of 72 outpatients with cerebral insufficiency. In this double-blind, placebo-controlled
   study, learning rate was measured at the start of
   the study, after 6 weeks, and again after 24 weeks.
   The results showed significant improvement in the
   test group but none in the placebo group.
◆ In a French study conducted in the following year
   led by H. Allain, 18 men and women, with an average age of 69.3 years and suffering from AAMI or
   slight AD, were compared for speed of information
   processing with a matched placebo group.[170] The
   test group performed significantly better than the
   control group.[171]

While the results from these three studies are generally positive, unfortunately other studies indicate that
ginkgo has little or no effectiveness on alleviating AD,
slowing AAMI, or improving memory. Even on the three
positive studies, we don't know whether the high drop-
out rate in the Le Bars study mentioned above (from 309
participants to 202) was because those people were experiencing no benefit, or for other reasons.

For most doctors and researchers alike, the verdict is
still out on ginkgo. Many questions remain to be an-
swered, such as when it is effective, how much should be

used, for how long, and for what specific disorders. We also have no information on how well commercially available ginkgo products match EGb 761. Thus, many other experts share our own view, namely that while ginkgo may have some limited efficacy in slightly retarding the progress of AD, there is no conclusive evidence that it works directly on improving AAMI, and almost certainly it is nowhere near as effective as PS.

Concern about possible adverse effects of *Ginkgo biloba* caused the Canadian Health Protection Branch to conduct hearings. Their conclusion was that, while toxic effects had been associated with the fruit, the fruit pulp, and the seed, *Ginkgo biloba* leaves and leaf extracts posed no health threat. The Canadian authorities do therefore allow ginkgo products to be sold, provided there is no direct or implied representation of therapeutic or pharmacological effect.[172] Since Canada is notoriously conservative in its assessments of the possible dangers of nutritional supplements, we feel that their acceptance of ginkgo represents an implicit endorsement of its safety. Moreover, Canada's findings are in line with our own view that, apart from the theoretical concerns associated with blood thinning noted above, ginkgo is a safe supplement for most people.

Ginkgo biloba is available in virtually every health-food, drug, food, and mass merchandise store in the United States as a dietary supplement. Like all nutritional supplements, it is not approved by the FDA as a medical treatment. Nevertheless, Americans spent more than $100 million on ginkgo supplements in 1997 alone, while a 1993 report indicated that Europeans spent the equivalent of about $500 million in U.S. dollars.[173]

After evaluating the body of research behind ginkgo, and especially the large study reported in *JAMA*, we conclude that ginkgo may perhaps be a useful adjunct to PS and the rest of the memory cure described in this book, but that it is most likely not a valuable supplement for alleviating AAMI on its own.

GINSENG

One of the most well-known herbs used for maintaining health and aiding people who are "mentally tired" is ginseng. An extensively researched herb, ginseng has been around for 3,000 years, used throughout Asian countries as a stimulant to restore flagging energy or to promote more energy. The root is sold in many forms: as a whole root, as a powdered or liquid extract, in granules for instant tea, and in tablets and capsules. It is broadly available in all retail outlets that sell supplements. Unfortunately, however, it is usually not possible to tell from which part of the plant specific extracts are made, but it is known that extracts made from the leaves are different from those made from the roots.

As with most herbs, for a number of years no one really knew why it worked. Then it was discovered that it contained 12 or 13 compounds called ginsenosides (fatty compounds of hydrogen and oxygen), which have a variety of contradictory effects. This may account for its wide-range popularity as a "cure" for a variety of remedies.

This variety of results is further aggravated by three additional problems:

◆ There are more than 200 different varieties of ginseng root and currently three major types of ginseng available in North America. We know of no way to differentiate between the potency or effectiveness of these significantly different supplements.

◆ Several recent investigations have shown that some products labeled ginseng contain little or no active ingredients.[174]

◆ Many vials of liquid ginseng may contain up to 34 percent alcohol, although many don't state that on the label, according to the Bureau of Alcohol, Tobacco and Firearms (BATF). Of 55 ginseng-containing vials tested by BATF in 1997, only seven were alcohol-free. While the alcohol may not be contraindicated for most people, it clearly confounds any benefits the ginseng may have. We therefore suggest that you check the ingredients and try to find a ginseng product that contains no alcohol.[175]

Given this variety of ginseng products, it is essentially impossible to know whether ginseng can help memory or not. On balance, however, we tend to the view that this supplement is going to add too little to the effect of PS and the balance of our memory cure to make it worthwhile.

CHOLINE

Choline and a variety of choline chemical analogs and alternatives such as phosphatidylcholine, cytidine diphosphate choline, choline chloride, and cytocholine, are precursors (and therefore necessary for the production of) the neurotransmitter *acetylcholine,* which is essential for proper transmission of impulses from cell to cell. Choline is also important for the making of cell membranes. Therefore, it is an important contributor to memory, and it is little wonder that mother's milk is high in choline, especially during the first few days after birth. In addition to helping improve the transmission of memory, choline also helps lower blood pressure and reduce cholesterol. Stress reduces the enzyme that is necessary to convert choline to acetylcholine.

Studies with both laboratory animals and a few humans indicate that choline may slightly improve memory performance. When rats were exposed to choline chloride supplementation, both prenatally (through the diet of the mothers) and postnatally, choline enhanced both working and reference memory, especially spatial memory capacity and precision in running mazes.[176] Rats with lesions of the nucleus basilis (a band of gray substance on the medulla oblongata, the connection between the spinal cord and the brain) showed higher concentrations of acetylcholine in the frontal cortex and improved memory acquisition and retention when given egg phosphatidylcholine combined with Vitamin B_{12}.[177] No well-designed studies of choline have been conducted on AAMI, and of the approximately 20 studies conducted on AD, most have been negative.

When cytocholine, involved in the biosynthesis of brain phospholipids and acetylcholine, was given to 24 elderly persons with memory deficits and without dementia, it improved word recall, immediate object recall, and delayed object recall.[178] A single dose of phosphatidylcholine resulted in significant improvement in explicit memory (in serial learning task) for 80 college students. Further analysis indicated that the improvement may have been due to improvement in the responses of slow learners rather than to a general effect[179]; hence, certain forms of choline may be more effective for slow learners than for others.

The brain is unable to make choline itself and must get it from our diets or from choline manufactured by the liver.[180] Some research shows that too little choline in the diet can cause a fatty buildup in the liver and liver dysfunction.[181] As we age, the brain becomes less efficient at manufacturing acetylcholine from choline. Lecithin, a byproduct of soybeans, is a major source of dietary choline, as are soybeans themselves. Other foods rich in choline include fish, seaweed, oatmeal, brown rice, black-eyed peas, garbanzo beans, split peas, lentils, cauliflower, cabbage, and kale.

At present there is no agreement as to how much choline a person needs. If you take choline or lecithin as a supplement, Vitamin B_5 is needed to convert choline into acetylcholine. Large doses of choline can occasionally cause gastric cramps, diarrhea, stiff neck, muscle tension, and headaches. These symptoms do not occur when taking lecithin.[182]

On the face of it, then, taking choline as a supplement might be helpful in augmenting the efficacy of PS. In practice, however, there is no need to ingest additional choline since the PS now manufactured by Lucas Meyer (i.e., LECI-PS™) already contains phosphatidylcholine as well.

The Need for Nutritional Supplements

The above three supplements are those most often mentioned in connection with improving memory. However, in addition to PS and possibly ginkgo and choline, it is vital that your body be properly nourished in all other respects. Thus in the following pages we shall discuss the main nutrients and nutritional supplements that will contribute to a healthy, balanced eating plan.

VITAMINS

All foods taken into the body must be broken down into their simplest components. Proteins become amino acids, carbohydrates are broken down into glucose (sugar), and fats into fatty acids. These processes require enzymes. That's where vitamins—organic substances that are required to regulate the functioning of the cells—come in. Essential to life, vitamins supply no energy, but rather assist enzymes by converting food into energy.

Although people on every continent have known for hundreds of years that certain foods seemed to prevent or cure certain diseases, it was not until 1911 that the first vitamin—thiamin, a B vitamin—was isolated in the lab. Since then, researchers have identified 13 additional vitamins.

Vitamins come in two varieties: fat-soluble (Vitamin A; beta-carotene, a precursor of Vitamins A, D, E; and Vitamin K) and water-soluble (the B vitamins and C). The body can store water-soluble vitamins for only a short time, but it can store fat-soluble vitamins in the liver and fatty tissue for many months. This means that it is easier to acquire toxic doses of stored fat-soluble vitamins than of water-soluble ones, since excess amounts of the latter are simply excreted.[183]

Deficiencies in almost any nutrient can cause changes in the functioning of the nervous system. There are some vitamins that are absolutely essential for proper memory function.

THE B VITAMINS: A COMPLEX FAMILY

Although we include a separate description of some of the more important B-complex vitamins, all the B vitamins are a team, each needing a certain amount of the other to perform its particular function well. A severe depletion in one (or too much of one over the others) causes a problem in the entire complex. If separate B-vitamin supplements are taken, they should always be

taken together, although up to two or three times more of
one B vitamin than another can be taken for a time to
counteract a particular disorder.[184] B-complex vitamins
are not as well absorbed as we age, so it is important to
have an adequate intake to maintain the health of the
nerves, produce energy in the body, and alleviate depression and anxiety. The B vitamins have an important impact on blood circulation, and a variety of other body
functions, all of which are necessary for the efficient operation of our brains. We should never forget that an unhealthy body is likely to interfere with the operation of
our minds and memories. Thus, we feel that taking a
group of B vitamins daily is a desirable part of our memory cure.

Vitamin B₁: The Nerve Vitamin

Vitamin B_1 (or thiamine) enhances circulation and assists in blood formation. It is important in the production
of hydrochloric acid, which is necessary for proper digestion. Because of its importance in the metabolism of
carbohydrates, the nervous system is particularly susceptible to thiamine deficiency.[185] According to Dr. James
Balch, author of a book called *Prescription for Natural
Healing,* thiamine "optimizes cognitive activity and
brain function."[186]

Although we don't need a lot of thiamine (1.5 milligrams for men, 1.1 milligrams for women), a thiamine
deficiency can show up as vision problems, irritability,
confusion, poor memory, sleep disturbance, fatigue, forgetfulness, mild depression, gastrointestinal disturbances, loss of appetite, nervousness, and general
weakness, among others in a long list of symptoms. It
was the absence of Vitamin B_1 in their diet that caused
the death of so many nineteenth-century sailors as a re-

sult of beriberi. Antibiotics, sulfa drugs, and oral contraceptives can decrease thiamine levels, and a high-carbohydrate diet also increases the need for this important vitamin.[187] Alcohol blocks the absorption of thiamine in the intestines, disrupts its storage in other bodily tissues, and interferes with its conversion into a form the body can use.[188]

Marinating meat in wine, soy sauce, or vinegar depletes between 50 and 75 percent of its thiamine content.[189] A group of enzymes called thiaminases, which destroy thiamine, have been found in raw fish (sushi), shellfish, some berries, Brussels sprouts, and red cabbage. Fortunately cooking renders these enzymes inactive.[190]

Thiamine is concentrated in brown rice, wheat germ and bran, whole grains, fortified cereals, nuts, and sunflower seeds. Other rich sources include poultry, roast pork, legumes, green peas, asparagus, broccoli, soybeans, kelp, and oatmeal.

The Helper Vitamin: Riboflavin

Riboflavin, or Vitamin B_2, is one of those vitamins that helps the body perform many tasks, including helping it change or release other nutrients. For instance, riboflavin helps change Vitamin B_6 and folic acid into forms the body can use. It also helps change the amino acid tryptophan into niacin, another essential B vitamin (see page 192).

The best way to get enough riboflavin is from foods, namely milk products (milk, yogurt, cheese, cottage cheese), egg whites, beef, pork, lamb, chicken, broccoli, and asparagus. Anyone who avoids dairy products, is a vegetarian, or is on a poorly balanced or low-calorie diet runs the risk of B_2 deficiency. Exercise increases the rate at which you excrete riboflavin; therefore, your need increases when you exercise. Although supplemental riboflavin is probably safe up to 100 milligrams daily (the RDA is 1.7 milligrams for men and 1.3 for women), large doses may cause kidney stones.[191]

Vitamin B₃: The Spark Plug Vitamin

Also known as niacin, Vitamin B₃ is necessary for at least 40 biochemical reactions that occur in the body.[192] There are two forms of this vitamin, niacinamide and nicotinic acid. Doctors often use high doses of the latter to lower blood cholesterol, since niacinamide does not have that effect. Niacin was the first substance ever shown to lower cholesterol and triglyceride levels, but because it is a nutrient, not a drug, it has not been widely promoted.[193]

Good sources of niacin include brewer's yeast, pork, the white meat of chicken and turkey, halibut, mackerel, salmon, tuna, tofu, cottage cheese, oats, peanuts (with skins better), cornflakes, kale, broccoli, carrots, tomatoes, and brown rice.

Vitamin B₅: The Anti-Stress Vitamin

Known also as pantothenic acid, Vitamin B₅ was discovered by Dr. Roger Williams more than thirty-five years ago and largely ignored for a number of years after. B₅ is required by all cells in the body including our brain cells. It plays a role in the production of the adrenal hormones, assists in the formation of antibodies, aids in the utilization of other vitamins, and helps convert food into energy.

Although most of us are likely to get a sufficient amount of pantothenic acid (4 to 7 milligrams daily), elderly persons who eat a limited diet and alcoholics are at risk of deficiency. Food processing, such as canning or freezing, destroys as much as 75 percent of the pantothenic acid in food. Sleeping pills, caffeine, and estrogen also destroy it.[194] Thus, if any of these conditions apply to you, you would be well advised to add supplemental Vitamin B_5 to your diet.

Good food sources are most fresh vegetables, and especially mushrooms, avocados, and broccoli, whole grains and bran, peanuts, cashews, legumes, soybeans, and pork.[195] As with most B vitamins, symptoms of deficiency include depression, fatigue, headache, and insomnia, all of which, of course, play havoc with your memory.

Vitamin B_6 Takes the Oscar for B Vitamins

B_6 deficiency has been linked to an extensive list of conditions and disorders. It easily wins an award for the vitamin with the largest number of benefits, and is believed to act as a partner for more than one hundred different enzymes.[196]

Vitamin B_6, sometimes called pyridoxine, is necessary for the production of hydrochloric acid and the absorption of fats and proteins, and is the key to the synthesis of several neurotransmitters. Without sufficient B_6 your body may not produce enough norepinephrine, serotonin, and dopamine.[197] B_6 also helps the body make red blood cells, stabilizes the nervous system, and is necessary for normal brain functioning. It aids in the absorption of Vitamin B_{12}, and it, too, helps convert tryptophan into niacin. The use of antidepressants, oral contraceptives, or estrogen therapy may increase the need for Vitamin B_6. Diuretics and cortisone drugs block its absorption.[198]

A 1992 Dutch study led by J. B. Diejen of the Free University in Amsterdam, investigated the effects Vitamin B_6 supplementation on mood and performance in 38 healthy men between the ages of 70 and 79 years. They were compared with 38 matched controls who received a placebo. Positive effects of Vitamin B_6 supplementation were found with respect to memory, especially long-term memory. Information storage was improved "modestly but significantly."[199]

Although actors would likely tell you that it is not possible to have too many Oscars, it is possible to get too much B_6, so don't start popping megadoses. Typically we only need 2 milligrams a day, so while you may need a little more B_6 as you age, the efficiency with which we utilize B_6 diminishes with age. Doses as low (or as high?) as 100 milligrams have been known to cause nerve damage. Overdoses can cause poor absorption of zinc and mask the symptoms of Vitamin B_{12} deficiency.

B_6 appears in many foods: nuts (especially Brazilian nuts and walnuts), sunflower seeds, poultry, fish, whole grains, salmon, oysters, soybeans, bananas, carrots, potatoes, avocados, broccoli, cauliflower, and ginger root. Freezing vegetables results in 57 to 77 percent reduction in their B_6 content.[200] Persons taking L-dopa (the precursor for the development of dopamine) for the treatment of Parkinson's disease should not take Vitamin B_6 except under the supervision of their physician.[201]

The Vitality Vitamin, B_{12}

Essential to the production of energy in the human body, Vitamin B_{12} also aids in digestion, absorption of foods, and the breakdown of carbohydrates and fats. It is needed to prevent anemia, which can rob the brain of oxygen. Better yet for our purposes, B_{12} aids in cell formation and cellular longevity, preventing nerve damage by manufacturing and maintaining the fatty sheath (called myelin) that covers and protects nerves. B_{12} is linked to the production of the neurotransmitter acetylcholine which, as we have said, is critical to memory and is increased by PS.

It's relatively rare that deficiencies of B_{12} occur, since most of us need only a daily dose of 2 micrograms of B_{12}, and the liver can store sufficient quantities to sustain the body's needs for three to five years. However, some deficiencies do occur, especially among older people who have difficulty with their digestion and may not be able to absorb B_{12} from their intestines. Untreated B_{12} deficiency can cause severe brain and nerve damage. Smokers, heavy drinkers, pregnant women, and people taking some potassium supplements, estrogen, sleeping pills, and anticoagulant drugs are also likely candidates for B_{12} deficiency.

One of the most noticeable and common symptoms of B_{12} deficiency is a "tingling" in the hands and feet. Having a low intake of B_{12} can also result in chronic fatigue, muscle weakness in the legs or arms, low appetite, depression, digestive disorders, memory loss, moodiness, nervousness, and certain neurological damage. Because the largest amounts of B_{12} are found in animal (notably beef) and fish products (sole, oysters, sardines, mackerel, and tuna) and milk and dairy products (Swiss cheese, cottage cheese, yogurt), vegetarians need to be especially careful.[202] The only vegetables that B_{12} is found in are soybeans and soy products and sea vegetables such as kelp, kombu, and nori. Other good sources of Vitamin B_{12} are brewer's yeast and eggs.[203] No matter how many good B_{12} foods you eat, however, a deficiency in the stomach's production of hydrochloric acid will impair the absorption of Vitamin B_{12}. Older people are particularly prone to diminished hydrochloric acid production.

Folic Acid: The Energy Vitamin

Also a vitamin of the B complex, folic acid is necessary for the body's utilization of sugar and for protein metabolism; hence, the body's energy relies on folic acid. While energy is not directly linked to memory, it is an adjunct to it. Without sufficient energy, we won't want to "be bothered" to exercise our minds or to continue to assimilate new information. And our memories will suffer.

The sugar from fresh fruit, vegetables (cooking destroys folic acid), and from grains enhances the absorption of folic acid, as do Vitamins B_{12} and C.[204] Good folic acid sources include: chicken livers, salmon, tuna, fresh deep-green leafy vegetables, broccoli, carrots, navy beans, beans (especially soybeans), barley, brown rice, sunflower seeds, sweet potatoes, apricots, cantaloupe, oranges, and orange juice.

THE ANTIOXIDANT VITAMINS

Aging processes, among them brain aging, are thought to be associated with free radical action. Thus, there is strong reason to believe that our memories, too, are adversely affected by free radicals. Certain nutrients consistently have been shown to prevent the oxidative damage caused by free radicals. When aged rats (24 months old) were given the equivalents of Vitamins C (ascorbate) and E (alpha-tocopherol) for five months daily, the antioxidant-treated rats exhibited significantly greater memory retention than control rats after only two months.[205]

A number of studies have investigated the mixed but intriguing results of the effects of antioxidants on Alzheimer's disease. Certainly, there is no implication yet that they cure the disease. But there may be interesting avenues for further research in this direction. Fortunately, however, you don't have to be either a rat or have Alzheimer's to benefit from the healthful benefits of antioxidants.

The Colorful Beta-Carotene

Not strictly a vitamin itself, beta-carotene is converted to Vitamin A in the intestinal wall. It has been shown to have powerful antioxidant effects and, as a result, to slow the effects of aging.[206] Evaluation of the dietary intake of 5,182 persons aged 55 to 95 years who were participants in the Rotterdam Study in The Netherlands showed that a lower intake of beta-carotene was associated with impaired cognitive function.[207] Such a lower intake is a reasonable possibility since antibiotics, laxatives, and some cholesterol-lowering drugs interfere with the absorption of the beta-carotene-induced Vitamin A.[208]

Given its powerful antioxidant qualities and its known effect on general mental acuity, we judge that beta-carotene should have some beneficial effect on memory. Beta-carotene is the best known of a family of substances called the *carotenoids,* which are found in the more deeply colored fruits and vegetables. Hence, you can get sufficient amounts of it by eating lots of these beautifully colored fruits and vegetables that your mother nagged you to eat: carrots, broccoli, kale, sweet potatoes, parsley, pumpkin, dark leafy greens, tomatoes, apricots, yellow squash, red bell peppers, pink grapefruit, cantaloupe, mangos, papayas, apricots, and peaches.

The Consummate Vitamin C

In addition to its service as an antioxidant, Vitamin C has been touted at one time or another for just about every illness known.[209] This remarkable vitamin helps promote healthy gums and teeth, maintain normal connective tissue, strengthen blood vessels, increase resistance to infection, and heal wounds. It aids in the production of antistress hormones. Among aged mice, after only three days of treatment, Vitamin C canceled the effects of scopolamine, a drug that interferes with acetylcholine in the brain and is used frequently in the lab to produce forgetting or amnesia.[210]

While no direct research applicable to humans is available, this is such an essential vitamin for all cellular functions that common sense tells us we should include it in the memory cure.

Stress, a habitually poor diet, illness, the use of oral contraceptives, and some medications all increase the body's need for Vitamin C, which is found in citrus fruits (grapefruit, lemons, and oranges), berries, red bell peppers, and green vegetables such as broccoli, Brussels sprouts, green peas, parsley, and watercress. It is also found in guavas, persimmons, cantaloupe, mangos, papayas, and pineapple.

VITAMIN E: THE SYNERGISTIC ANTIOXIDANT

Vitamin E is important in the maintenance of cell membranes and tissue repair. It improves circulation, helps in the formation of red blood cells, and helps prevent the aggregation of platelets, disk-shaped components of the blood that promote clotting. Vitamin E enhances immune function and, as an antioxidant, it protects other fat-soluble vitamins from destruction by oxygen. A deficiency of Vitamin E may result in the destruction of nerves and the reduction of memory.[211] And a recent study sponsored by the National Institute on Aging suggests that very large doses of Vitamin E (2,000 i.u. daily) may have a small beneficial impact on AD.

There is also some evidence that, as antioxidants, Vitamins E and C work synergistically, becoming more powerful together. While Vitamin E scavenges for free radicals in cell membranes, Vitamin C attacks the free radicals in the body's fluids.[212]

Some forms of inorganic iron (ferrous sulfate) destroy Vitamin E, so iron supplements should be taken at a different time of the day from Vitamin E supplements. Organic forms (ferrous gluconate or ferrous fumarate) leave Vitamin E intact.[213]

Persons on very low-fat diets need to be aware that fat ingestion is important to Vitamin E intake and metabolism.

Vitamin E is found in cold-pressed vegetable oils, leafy greens, legumes, soybeans and soybean oil, olive oil, whole grains, brown rice, kelp, milk, oatmeal, sweet potatoes, peanuts and peanut butter, and sunflower seeds. If you are taking an anticoagulant or any other medication that affects blood clotting, you shouldn't take Vitamin E supplements; they are themselves anticoagulants, and the result of the combination might cause problems.[214]

We realize that this listing of vitamins may seem a bit daunting when each of them is discussed individually. However, in practice, all you need to do is take one good multivitamin daily (in the quantities recommended by a reputable manufacturer) and if necessary augment it with an additional dose of beta-carotene. If you do that, your body will be getting all the vitamins it needs to optimize its health, energy, and, derivatively, its memory.

The Memory Minerals

Minerals are one of the six nutrients our body needs, the others being vitamins, water, protein, carbohydrates and fats. According to orthomolecular physicians Abram Hoffer and Morton Walker, minerals are actively engaged in "strengthening the nervous system, normalizing the heartbeat, providing energy, improving thinking power, overcoming fatigue, building a dynamic memory, and sparking our other metabolic processes."[215] Minerals come in two kinds. Major minerals are needed in large amounts, and trace minerals in minute quantities (they may be toxic in larger amounts).

Again, for the most part, these minerals have not been individually found to affect memory directly except, in some cases, where serious deficiencies may impair memory. However, they are vital to your overall health, especially if you are over 50. Therefore, we shall cover them here briefly.

CALCIUM

Most of us already know that we need calcium—the most abundant mineral in our bodies—for healthy bones and teeth. What you may not know is that it is essential for the development of normal nerve tissue, to regulate heartbeat, and for blood clotting. Calcium is absorbed from the intestine by a process requiring Vitamin D. Too much fat, oxalic acid (found in spinach, kale, rhubarb, cocoa, and chocolate), and phytic acid (found in grains) results in calcium not being absorbed.[216] This is one of the reasons that chocolate milk, so beloved by children and so popular in school cafeterias, is not really a healthy drink.

Calcium may also have an effect on mood, but the process is complex. A little stimulates the nerves and elevates the mood, but too much can depress nerve activity and mood.[217] We do not know exactly how, or even whether, it affects memory. However, we do know that calcium is essential for a healthy body (including the avoidance of osteoporosis), and we therefore urge you to make sure you take enough of it.

High protein intake, alcohol, and caffeine make calcium less available to the body. Fiber binds calcium, so it is best to avoid eating your calcium with high-fiber meals. Vitamin D, magnesium, and boron are essential to the absorption of calcium, so if you take calcium and vitamin supplements, take them at the same time.[218] Consumption of white flour and soft drinks, which are high in phosphorus, lead to increased excretion of calcium. Heavy exercising hinders calcium intake, but moderate exercise promotes it.[219]

Excellent sources of calcium are kelp, milk, cheese, (especially ricotta), yogurt, tofu, salmon and sardines with bones, and dried figs. Other good sources include corn tortillas, leafy green vegetables, parsley, watercress, broccoli, okra, soybeans, and chickpeas (also known as garbanzo beans), Brazil nuts, and seeds (sunflower, pumpkin, and squash).

MAGNESIUM

Magnesium, too, is an essential mineral. It is an important catalyst in enzyme activity, especially that involved in energy production. Magnesium also plays a role in regulating the stability of cell membranes. A deficiency of magnesium interferes with the transmission of muscle and nerve impulses, slowing down the processing of memories and other messages. As we grow older, for some of us our circulation slows down. Magnesium minimizes the negative effects of reduced blood flow, assuring a good supply of nutrients to brain cells. Magnesium deficiency is often at the root of many cardiovascular problems. It has been touted as an antistress mineral because a magnesium deficiency can cause nervousness, irritability, and depression.[220] As we have emphasized before, depression interferes with effective memory.

Unfortunately, many heart drugs, such as digitalis or digoxin, reduce the amount of magnesium in the body. Therefore, if you are on these drugs, we urge you not to take a magnesium supplement without first consulting your doctor to see if you *are* one of those who might need it.

Magnesium also fights calcification (calcium buildup) in neurons. Calcification kills neurons and has been implicated in some studies of patients with Alzheimer's disease. Magnesium enhances the immune system and prevents osteoporosis. Important for the conversion of blood sugar (glucose) into energy, it reduces the risk of diabetes by improving glucose tolerance (poor glucose tolerance often precedes the development of diabetes).

Rich food sources of magnesium are dairy products, seafood, a number of fruits (apples, avocados, bananas, apricots, peaches, cantaloupe, grapefruit), blackstrap molasses, brown rice, green leafy vegetables, kelp, whole grains, soy products (soybeans, tofu), Brazil nuts, filberts, and sunflower seeds. A diet rich in fats and protein, the intake of fat-soluble vitamins, and foods high in oxalic acid (almonds, cocoa, spinach, tea) all decrease magnesium absorption.[221]

Men need 350 milligrams of magnesium daily and women, 280 milligrams. Calcium and magnesium should be taken in a ratio of 1:1, since too much or too little magnesium in relation to calcium interferes with the body's absorption of calcium. Losses of magnesium occur whenever you take a diuretic, or drink excess coffee, tea, or alcohol.[222]

If you eat a diet high in magnesium or take supple-

MEMORY MOMENT _____

" G od gave us memory so that we might have roses in December."

—J. M. Barrie, British playwright and author of *Peter Pan*.

ments, you should be aware of the fact that some over-the-counter products also contain magnesium and can raise your level high enough to produce diarrhea. These products include Maalox, Mylanta, Phillips' milk of magnesia, De-Gel, Bayer Plus, and Bufferin.[223]

ZINC, AN IMPORTANT TRACE MINERAL

Did your mother ever tell you to eat your fish, using that phrase that is an integral part of mothers' vocabularies worldwide: "because it's good for you"? Possibly she added that fish was "brain food." Well, she may have been right. Fish, especially oysters (six cooked medium-sized Eastern oysters provide about 76 milligrams of zinc), herring, clams, and tuna, all contain high levels of zinc. Deficiencies of this trace mineral may be involved in concentration and short-term memory deficits, although most of the studies showing that have been conducted using laboratory animals, primarily rats and rhesus monkeys. For instance, in several studies zinc-deficient rats showed a loss of working (short-term) memory for learning a 17-arm radial maze when compared to adequately nourished rats.[224]

Zinc is present in all bodily organs, and is the key to many physical processes. It is believed to help regulate chemical communications between brain cells, and is vital to the activity of many of the body's enzymes. Zinc-containing enzymes are involved in numerous metabolic processes, particularly cell replication. Zinc is important to proper functioning of the immune system. It also helps the body better absorb Vitamin A, and is necessary for the proper maintenance of Vitamin E levels.

One sign of zinc deficiency is lack of taste and resulting lack of appetite, often common in elderly people who don't eat enough foods high in zinc and also don't absorb zinc as well as they did when they were younger. Pregnant women are at risk for deficiency, as are vegetarians, because the fiber and other substances in many plant foods interfere with the absorption of zinc. Drugs such as tetracycline, cortisone, and diuretics can also interfere with zinc absorption. A Norwegian study showed that the quantity of zinc was significantly lower in the semen of smokers than nonsmokers, which might contribute to reproductive failure or poor fetal development.[225]

In addition to fish, other good sources of zinc are wheat bran, wheat germ, lamb, chicken, most beans—especially black-eyed peas, garbanzo beans, lentils, and green peas—brown rice, oatmeal, and soy products. Some zinc is found in cranberry juice, applesauce, peanut butter, eggs, and cooked spinach. Be alerted, however, that mega-amounts of zinc, such as you might get if you double-up on vitamin/mineral supplements while eating an adequate amount of dietary zinc, can inhibit calcium absorption if dietary calcium is already low.[226]

The RDA for men is 15 milligrams and 12 milligrams for women. Doses in excess of those amounts can adversely affect the immune system and prevent the absorption of copper, iron, and calcium. On the other hand, Dr. Richard Wood, chief of the Mineral Bioavailability Laboratory at the USDA Human Nutrition Research Center on Aging at Tufts University in Boston, told the newsletter *Bottom Line Health* that seniors who are careful to get enough calcium (1,200 milligrams per day) may be depleting their bodies of zinc, since that much calcium can block zinc absorption. If you're taking calcium, ask your doctor about adding a 10-milligram zinc supplement to your daily regimen, suggests Dr. Wood.[227]

If supplemental zinc is taken—with a doctor's advice—copper supplements (one-tenth the zinc dosage) should be taken as well.[228] Another good reason not to overdose on zinc is that scientists have found higher content than normal of aluminum, zinc, and other metals in the brain tissue of people with Alzheimer's disease. It is not yet clear whether they are part of the cause of the disease or built up in the brain as a result of it, says the Alzheimer's Disease Education and Referral Center of the National Institute on Aging, the leading agency for Alzheimer's research.

BORON KEEPS THE ELECTRICITY GOING

One of the reasons fruits and nuts are so good for your brain is that they are high in boron, a trace mineral that affects the body's ability to metabolize minerals and increase the electrical activity of the brain. The lower your intake of boron, the more sluggishly your brain reacts and the less alert you are.

One of the leading scientists studying the effects of boron is research psychologist James G. Penland of the U.S. Department of Agriculture's Agricultural Research Service at Grand Forks, North Dakota. While boron has yet to be recognized as an essential nutrient for humans, Dr. Penland found that in several studies with healthy older men and women when low boron intake (0.25 milligrams boron/200 kcal/day) was compared to high intake (3.25 milligrams), low boron intake resulted in a significant increase in the proportion of low-frequency brain activity and a decrease in the proportion of higher-frequency activity. The effect, measured by a spectral analysis of electroencephalographic information, is similar to that often observed as a result of general malnutrition and heavy metal toxicity. Low boron intake also resulted in significantly poorer performances on tasks emphasizing manual dexterity, eye-hand coordination, attention, perception, encoding, and short-term memory and long-term memory.[229]

Boron is also necessary for the metabolism of calcium, magnesium, and phosphorus, and is needed in trace amounts for healthy bones. Although most people are not deficient in boron, elderly people who have a problem with calcium absorption may need to take a supplement of 2 to 3 milligrams per day.[230]

Where do you find boron in foods? An old adage may help you. Remember "an apple a day keeps the doctor away"? Apples, pears, peaches, and grapes are especially good sources of boron, as are nuts, legumes, cauliflower, broccoli, and green leafy vegetables, especially kale.

IRON

Iron is essential for making hemoglobin, the red substance in blood that carries oxygen to your brain cells. Hence it is essential for memory maintenance. Although it is the mineral found in the largest amounts in the blood, iron is widely distributed through the body. Iron is required for a healthy immune system and for energy production.[231]

Iron deficiency anemia typically occurs with an inadequate diet, but iron also leaves the body through blood loss, which is why women who still menstruate may be prone to deficiencies. Intestinal bleeding, repeated pregnancy, chronic diarrhea, a diet high in phosphorus, poor digestion, long-term illness, prolonged use of antacids, strenuous exercise, and heavy perspiration are other conditions that can rob the body of iron. Iron is more readily absorbed when eaten or taken with Vitamin C. Caffeine decreases its absorption, as do excessive amounts of Vitamin E and zinc.[232]

Iron is found in eggs, fish (especially clams and oysters), red meat, and poultry. Other good sources include blackstrap molasses, fortified cereals, avocados, beets, kelp, kidney and lima beans, brewer's yeast, prune juice, green leafy vegetables, asparagus, oatmeal, tofu, soybeans, pumpkins and pumpkin seeds, and sunflower seeds. Experts have very controversial ideas on whether or not you need iron reserves and some studies suggest such reserves may increase the risk of heart attacks; hence, iron supplements should never be taken except on the advice of a physician who has determined your need of them from a blood test.[233]

SELENIUM

A trace mineral discovered in 1817 by Swedish chemist Jons Jakob Berzelius, selenium detoxifies heavy metals such as lead, mercury, and cadmium, which are poisonous to the brain and upset its chemistry. Even small amounts of these toxic metals can interfere with thinking and memory. Research in the 1950s discovered that selenium is absorbed into the molecules of an enzyme called *glutathione peroxidase,* which is essential for the protection of red blood cells and of cell membranes. A powerful antioxidant, selenium deactivates free radicals and makes Vitamin E more effective. Selenium increases the production of antibodies that fight infection and strengthens the immune system.[234] For all these reasons, selenium probably has a salutary impact on memory.

Foods high in selenium include whole grain breads and cereals, Brazil nuts, scallops, wheat germ, bran, and barley, provided they are grown in selenium-rich soil, and this can be a problem. Selenium originates in soil, where it is absorbed by growing plants. More is not better in the case of selenium, since at high levels it can be toxic.

In 1989 the Food and Nutrition Board of the National Research Council set the RDA at 70 micrograms for men and 55 micrograms for women. Most of us easily get that much if our diet includes tuna, herring, shellfish, dairy products, asparagus, mushrooms, onions, and Brazil nuts.[235]

Is Food Medicine?

In this chapter we have seen how something normally considered a food—nutrients—can also have therapeutic purposes, especially when taken in larger amounts than might normally be consumed. The boundaries between nutrients and drugs gets fuzzier with each passing day, as evidenced by a recent article titled "Food as Medicine" in the newsletter *Women's Health Watch* published by Harvard Medical School. Two randomized, controlled clinical trials demonstrated that eating plans may be sensible alternatives to drug treatment. They show that we can develop new patterns of eating that can serve us for a lifetime of good health.[236]

The general point here is that a sensibly controlled diet that contains a balance of the major food groups, sufficient fiber, and those special foods we have listed above to add specific memory-beneficial supplements, is necessary to maintain all aspects of good health, including the health of our minds and memories.

Thus, while this is not a diet or general health book, we would like to emphasize that a healthy diet full of a variety of foods is one of the best ways to enhance the effectiveness of your PS supplement, to heighten the production of neurotransmitters important for neuronal communication, and to maintain your general health in order to avoid memory-robbing illnesses.

For most vitamins and minerals, natural foods are better and safer than supplements because they make it more difficult for an undesirable or even toxic buildup to occur. They also make your meals more interesting. Don't get stuck in the rut of the same old foods every day because they're easy to fix. They may not be so healthy for your body. Reinforce your mental processes: improve your diet!

8

Dealing with Stress

How does stress harm our memory?

Stress is necessary

◆

Managing stress

◆

Keeping things in perspective

❖

Every one of us, in the course of our daily lives, faces stress. It is unavoidable. Moreover, up to a point, it is also good for us. Few of us would do our best work—or do it on time—if we were not up against a stressful deadline. The extra adrenaline we get from knowing that a task *must* be finished by a set time, even if we know that the deadline is artificial, gives us the incentive we need to complete the task. There are few of us who haven't put something off "to the very last minute."

Then there are the high-stress jobs many of us choose. They are the ones with lots of deadlines, and often deadlines which are neither arbitrary nor trivial. There is nothing unimportant or delayable about an air-traffic controller's job, making sure that the planes landing don't crash into each other. Sometimes, as in stock trading for instance, each "deadline" is only seconds away. If you don't make the buy right now, the opportunity will be permanently lost. That naturally adds to the stress.

One of the observable facts about high-stress jobs is that they tend to be better paid than low-stress ones. The reason is obvious: they require an unusual degree of competence and calmness, and there are not too many people who wittingly take or choose a high-stress job. And yet, once you are employed, nearly all jobs seem to carry with them relatively high levels of stress. People in the high-paying, supposedly high-stress jobs get used to them, become inured to the stress, and don't feel its negative effects all that much. Conversely, people in the low-stress, lower-paying jobs develop spats with their co-workers, or feel pressured by their supervisors, and consequently feel more stress than they bargained for. In a sense, the high-income earners are paid for stress they don't face; the others are uncompensated for stress they do face.

Why, we may ask, is this? How does it happen that stress seems to level out?

The reason is that stress is something we do to ourselves, not usually something forced upon us by our employers or the circumstances of our employment. We generate stress by worrying too much about the components of our jobs, our competitors, our subordinates. And, of course, we worry too much about whether we're performing adequately. As a result of this constant set of worries, we constantly experience stress.

Thus, on the one hand, we evidently crave a certain amount of stress and are motivated by it, while, on the other, there is no doubt that stress lowers our capacity to remember, and, by the time we reach a certain age, probably contributes to AAMI.

For aging people, a major stress is the worry about their changing physical condition. As they age, people ask themselves, "Will I remember enough to continue to play bridge?" "Am I starting to lose my mind?" "Will I become a doddering old fool?" With a population of almost 65 million otherwise healthy people over the age of 50, these questions add up to a whole lot of needless frustration. If you're one of those persons, rest assured *The Memory Cure* can help you prevent the adverse effects of that stress.

Environmental, economic, and social stressors are also high on the list of memory debilitators. Memory experts tell us that, in the brain, repeated stress, disorganization, and lack of concentration all have a negative influence on our ability to remember important facts. This may be one of the key reasons that people in pressure-packed jobs complain of memory problems no matter what their age.

How Does Stress Harm Our Memory?

Almost any kind of stressful situation where strong emotions are aroused can interfere with your ability to learn and remember. By distracting us, worry also interferes with learning and memory. Young adults in their twenties reported that most of their memory problems occurred when they were under stress.[237] In a laboratory situation, people who are generally more anxious about life tend to do worse on memory tests than people with a low general-anxiety level.[238]

Chronic stress depletes the neurotransmitter norepinephrine, so important in laying down memories. It also lowers blood sugar, a situation particularly dangerous to the brain since it uses more than 20 percent of the body's blood sugar while at rest, and even more while engaging in mental tasks. Our bodies naturally generate a certain amount of stress hormones daily. We need them to survive, but during periods of particular stress the amount of many of these hormones increases. When they increase, they shut down the transport of sugar (glucose) into brain cells, which, as all cells do, depend on glucose for energy. There are different concentrations of receptors for glucocorticoids in different parts of the brain, and one of these that is particularly vulnerable is the hippocampus, which, as we have already learned, is a critical site in the memory process.

An example of the profound effects of stress is a study in which the growth rate of the offspring of pregnant rats stressed at the tenth or nineteenth gestational day was shown to be lower and their death rate much higher than that of the offspring of nonstressed control rats. As adults, the offspring of the stressed mothers exhibited learning and memory impairments. This study suggests that stress to the mothers resulted in hormonal changes and subsequent dysfunctions in the development of the nervous system of their offspring.[239]

Stress increases the body's need for proteins and for carbohydrates, the latter by releasing a brain chemical called neuropeptide Y. Stress increases the loss of Vitamin C and zinc. It impairs memories that track our everyday activities and accelerates several biological markers of aging, including age-related neuronal damage.

Restraining rats, a particularly stressful situation for them, caused atrophy of dendrites in the neurons of the hippocampus. This change in synaptic function was accompanied by specific cognitive deficits in spatial learning and memory. It could be relieved somewhat by the neurotransmitter serotonin, which is created in humans when we relax deeply or sleep.[240]

Our worries about loss of memory are aggravated by even the most casual slips of memory, but those very worries themselves erode confidence, which then leads to more anxiety and stress. A debilitating cycle begins. Soon you're too anxious and have too little confidence to work on your memory abilities. You decide your memory is "going," and that you therefore no longer have the tools for intellectual challenge. As a result, in a classic self-fulfilling prophecy, you ignore or avoid just the kind of mental stimulation that could keep your memory skills active. You give up too easily on a memory task that you might have accomplished if you had persevered a little longer. Proof positive, you think to yourself, that your memory truly is slipping. And you feel a little worse and lose a little more confidence.

It is a strange paradox that the more you worry about losing your memory, the more likely you are to have poorer and poorer memory. One of the simplest ways to reduce your stress and improve your memory is by having the confidence that you *can* remember.

Cognitive loss, and the resulting social embarrassment, can also lead to lowered self-esteem, withdrawal from friends and family, and may exacerbate the severe depression that is, unfortunately, all too common among older people. Untreated depression alone can be a definite factor in memory loss; fortunately, the effects can often be reversed when the depression is treated.

Stress Is Necessary

Most of us think we have too much stress in our lives and that it would be nice to have no stress, but this is not true. We need a certain amount of stress to accomplish our life activities—and even to remember. The problem is that we inherited from our ancient ancestors only two ways to handle stress, both physical: fight or flight. During those early cave-dwelling days, handling stress was simple: As soon as the crisis loomed, our ancestors either killed the enemy (usually a threatening animal), or they ran and saved their lives. In both cases, the activity used up the extra sugar and other chemicals that the stress had created. Then, having escaped the danger, they could then relax and calm down. These ways of handling stress helped them survive so successfully that they passed the "skill" on to us, through generations and generations of their descendants.

Today our stressors are not so easily confronted or escaped. No one lives a risk-free life. Busy lives, constant media exposure to threatening events, and the pressures of successfully learning to combine job, marriage, and family are likely to keep us in fight or flight mode 24 hours a day. We're plopped right down in the middle of stressful situations where fleeing is not an alternative and fighting is not acceptable. Some of our bosses would like us to believe that becoming a workaholic is the best, maybe even the only, way to survive and be a successful employee. Our adrenal glands work overtime to continually release epinephrine, norepinephrine, and other stress hormones into our system to help us cope, but we have no easy way to work off our stress and use up the extra chemicals.

Often, even the anticipation of future stress is stressful. When a group of 14 healthy elderly adults was involved in a nonstressful (attentional) task and a stressful one (public speaking), the stressful one significantly decreased memory performance. Dividing the group into "responders" and "nonresponders" highlighted the fact that the responders increased their cortisol levels 60 minutes before the actual stressor, whereas nonresponders increased their cortisol levels only 25 minutes before, suggesting that the anticipation of stress may have played a more significant role in the stress-induced memory deficits.[241] This suggests that we need to learn to combat the effects of stress when stressors are first presented to us rather than after the situation has passed, although that is also a good time to use stress management techniques to "recover." It is also of interest that PS has been shown in multiple studies to decrease elevations in cortisol associated with stress to the body.

We may think we've learned ways to unwind and thereby cope with stress, or at least recover. To this end, we consume alcoholic drinks to help us relax; we throw temper tantrums to work off our rage; we overwork to deal with the stress-producing problems of the day; we overeat because it satisfies our psyches; we smoke cigarettes; and some of us take either street or prescription drugs (or both). And those behaviors may seem to restore or reassure us temporarily, but, of course, they are actually dead-end streets when it comes to resolving our stress and leading a more relaxed life.

Our society constantly reinforces the message that relaxation, or time off, is not something we should enjoy every day—we have to postpone it until our once-a-year vacation. That's just not so. On the contrary, we're here to advise you that there are lots of ways you can add relaxation to your life while you're waiting for that vacation. You've probably heard of the fictional boss who is pleased to announce, "I don't feel stress, I give it!" Well, you too can learn to live with and even enjoy stress (although you don't necessarily have to mete it out). The key is not to try to avoid stress, but to change your perspective and learn to manage it.

Managing Stress

Learning to manage your stress is actually a decision-making process. First you have to decide you want to develop coping skills that help you transform stress into something else. Then you have to find the stress techniques that work best for you, since not all techniques work well for all people.

Yoga, stretching, walking outdoors, breathing, meditation, t'ai chi, and visualizing oneself in a relaxing setting are some of the varied techniques that people use to help them relax. Videotapes are available to teach you yoga, meditation, and t'ai chi, although you might enjoy participating in a class at your local YMCA.

One of the easiest of all the stress-busting techniques is to stop whatever it is you are doing and take a few minutes to breathe deeply. Yes, breathe. A deeper, slower rate of breathing contributes to calmness, deeper thinking, and better metabolism, while shallow, fast breathing can lead to superficial thinking and impulsive behavior.[242]

All stress management experts include changing the way you breathe in their repertoire of stress management techniques. It's so simple and is something you do all the time anyway. Depending on the stress expert, breathing can range from simply taking more deep breaths (inhaling through your nose and exhaling fully through your mouth) to five or ten minutes of diaphragmatic or "belly" breathing, to 50 to 60 minutes (or more) of yoga breathing combined with meditation. Don't let that scare you.

Anytime you stop and focus fully on your breathing, even for a few deep breaths, you turn off those raging thoughts that are driving you mad. To make those extra deep breaths you're now going to take several times a day more effective, as you inhale, say to yourself, "Relax." As you exhale, say, "Let go," and feel your shoulders actually let go. Most of us have grown so used to carrying the weight of the world around on our shoulders every day, we aren't even aware of it.

Did you know that your body is designed to discharge 70 percent of its toxins through breathing? Taking time to take those deep breaths means your kidneys and other systems don't have to work so hard.

◆ **Give Yourself Permission to Daydream.** We know your teachers and parents may have scolded you for daydreaming as a child, but daydreams do serve a purpose, so take time to daydream. According to Steven Jay Lynn, professor of psychology at State University of New York in Binghamton, daydreams can help us organize our lives, develop goals, lower stress, and make it easier to cope with problems. They are not idle pastimes, but rather ways we reveal our hopes and fears to ourselves and explore options in our lives.[243]

Whatever you already do to become physically quiet—listening to music, looking out a window, staring straight ahead—can become an effective stress management technique if you add the element of mental focus, says Dr. Kenneth R. Pelletier, a longevity expert with Stanford University Medical School in Palo Alto. As you take a few minutes to gaze out the window, choose a sound, word, image, or even your breath to focus on. Each time you notice your attention wandering away from it, return your mind to that focus. Even a few minutes a day of this kind of focused relaxation can decrease levels of stress hormones.[244]

MEMORY MOMENT

BELLY BREATHING

Belly breathing, one of the most effective ways of breathing, is an excellent way to reduce stress, banish negative thoughts, and clear our bodies of toxins when done consciously. Most of us breathe shallowly, moving our chest out and our shoulders up. Look in the mirror and observe which way you're breathing. What moves when you breathe, your shoulders or your abdomen?

You can help your body relax by deliberately switching from shoulder to belly breathing. Now each inhalation begins with the expansion of the abdominal muscles (imagine your abdomen is a balloon filling with air), which draws down and flattens the diaphragm, a large, dome-shaped sheet of muscle that separates the chest cavity from the abdomen. By increasing the size of the lower chest cavity, the lungs and rib area can expand. Your chest muscles—not your shoulders—move as your lungs fill with air. In exhalation the reverse occurs. The abdominal muscles contract. The upward movement of the diaphragm squeezes the lungs into the upper part of the chest, allowing them to expel large quantities of air, making it easier for you to take in more air with your next inhalation.

◆ **Use Imagery Exercises.** One of the most effective ways to relax is to close your eyes, focus inward, and *use your imagination* to gradually allow your body to become deeply comfortable. Many people have used the power of imagination to reduce anxiety, decrease chronic muscle tension and pain, to speed healing and recovery from surgery, and to ease sleep problems and many more conditions.

There are many such imagery exercises in popular stress management and wellness books. In case you don't have any of those, you can follow the technique below. You might want to have a friend read it to you, or better yet, record it in your own voice, pausing where we have inserted dots to allow yourself time to let go. The whole exercise should take you from 15 to 25 minutes. Do not rush through it in less time.

The more you practice the exercise, the more you will make it your own, and the more quickly your body will relax each time you do the exercise. If you make a tape, do not listen to it while driving. As you get more experienced, you may notice that you lose the sense that you have legs and feet. This is simply a signal that you are becoming deeply relaxed. If it worries you at first, just wiggle your hands or feet slightly to reassure yourself and to also notice what happens when you do. After awhile, you'll realize that you still have all arms and legs intact.

To begin the exercise settle back in your chair, lie down on a couch, or otherwise get yourself in a comfortable position that you can maintain for the duration of the exercise.

Take a deep breath in through your nose . . . and as you let it out through your mouth, with a big sigh . . . allow your eyes to close . . . Take another deep breath . . . and as you exhale, let it carry all the tension from your body . . . Take a moment to focus on any discomfort anywhere and shift your position to get more comfortable . . .

Turn your attention inward and begin to pay attention to any sensations you notice . . . Find the place in your body that seems the most tense . . . Tighten that muscle and hold, hold, hold it for a few seconds . . . Now let go and allow it to relax . . . Check around to find another tight muscle . . . Tighten it even more for a few seconds . . . Then let go and feel the release . . .

Check your breathing and feel yourself let go even more . . . as you imagine your breath carrying toxins out of your body. See them flowing out . . . feel your chest moving in and out . . . expanding and releasing . . . So calm . . . so comfortable . . .

Now direct your attention to the top of your head and imagine a golden sun or ball of light above you . . . Open a pathway from the top of your head to the tips of your toes and allow the golden warmth to enter your body . . . It feels silky smooth . . . and flows effortlessly down and through your body to the tips of your toes like golden honey . . . Focus on your feet and allow them to fill with the golden, warming energy . . .

Take all the time you need to feel your feet relax and become limp and warm . . . Gradually let that feeling of warmth and relaxation extend upward into your calves and lower legs . . . Get a sense of them filling with the warmth . . . as you become more and more comfortable . . . more and more relaxed . . . Your feet and lower legs are relaxed and heavy . . . warm and comfortable . . .

Now allow the warmth and relaxation to extend into your thighs and upper legs . . . Take all the time you need . . . to let your feet and legs go completely limp . . . Toes and feet . . . calves and thighs . . . all warm and comfortable . . . deeply relaxed . . .

Let the warmth and relaxation continue to rise into

your lower body . . . Feel the relaxation there . . . as your buttock lets go . . . The warmth eases and relaxes your lower back . . . the small of your back . . . and your abdomen becomes comfortable . . . You may notice your stomach muscles sagging a little as they relax their hold . . . And you may be interested to realize that it is so easy . . . for your breathing to become deeper and deeper . . . more and more comfortable . . . Simply allow all the muscles of your lower torso to experience a feeling of warmth . . . and heaviness . . . relaxing even more deeply.

Let that feeling of deep relaxation and warm energy spread fully through your chest and into the muscles of your upper back . . . flowing down into your shoulders and upper arms . . . Let your shoulders and arms go completely limp . . . Upper arms relaxing . . . becoming warm and heavy . . . lower arms relaxing . . . as the golden warmth flows into your hands and fingers . . . All the tension flowing right out of your fingertips . . . The muscles of your arms, and hands, and fingers feeling more and more relaxed . . . Taking all the time you need . . . to feel your arms and hands relax and become limp and warm . . . feeling calm . . . and relaxed . . . through your upper body.

Now let the muscles of your neck relax . . . and allow the feeling of relaxation to spread upward into your cheek and face muscles . . . as you let your jaw go . . . Jaw muscles and lips relaxing . . . ears letting go . . . All the muscles around the sides and back of your head fully relaxing . . . Now pay special attention to your forehead . . . feel the muscle there . . . and let it go . . . Allow the muscles in your scalp to relax . . . Let yourself feel how relaxed and comfortable your face and head

are . . . smooth and relaxed . . . just the right temperature for you . . .

    With your entire body deeply relaxed . . . you become
aware that you feel only a pleasant overall sensation of
warmth . . . and heaviness . . . peace . . . and comfort
. . . Know that you can return to this peaceful state
whenever you want . . . Take a few moments to concentrate on this feeling . . . as your body stores the sense
memory . . . so that later you can retrieve it . . . and
return to this deep state of relaxation . . .

    Each time you practice, know that you will relax
more deeply, more effortlessly, more comfortably . . .

    When you feel ready . . . in your own good time . . .
gently bring your awareness back to this room. Wiggle
your fingers and toes . . . make small movements . . .
and whenever you are ready, open your eyes, feeling
good and fine, feeling fully alive and filled with energy.

◆ **Appreciate Yourself.** A major step you can take
to reduce your stress is to be nice to yourself. Unfortunately that sounds easier than it is. Think about it. What
do most of us do when we mess up or can't remember
something? Smack ourselves on the head and say something like, "I'm so stupid," or "What a dummy!" That
might be okay if we stopped there, although we can't
in good conscience even advocate that small amount of
negativity toward oneself. Some of us go on with a tirade
of name-calling and statements that suggest a transformation from negativity into a full-blown self-loathing.

    The negative things we say about ourselves definitely
influence the way we feel during the day. Changing those
negative thoughts into more positive, loving ones is
called *cognitive therapy* and the first step involves listening to yourself—something most of us don't do often

enough. Once you've really heard the things you say, you can change them, or reprogram yourself to say more positive things. There are several ways you can do this.

A psychologist friend of ours told about writing a positive note to her patient on a 3" × 5" card that the patient could carry in her purse, and always have available to read. As they progressed in therapy, the patient began to write her own loving notes to herself. One friend writes positive notes to and about himself on yellow Post-it notes and puts them on his bathroom mirror, in the kitchen, and on the walls or furniture in other locations in his house where he frequently stands or sits. Daily he reinforces good thoughts about himself, and we think this is at least part of the reason why he's one of the most good-natured people we know.

◆ **Sleep Longer.** Another good way to reduce stress is to be certain that you get enough sleep. Many of us are sleep-deprived. Stress and anxiety can go round and round. High stress levels can keep you from falling asleep easily. Not falling asleep can cause you even more concern or anxiety. According to Stanley Coren, author of *Sleep Thieves*,[245] 13 million Americans take a prescription sleep medication, even though these same medications are a major cause of insomnia. They may cause you to fall asleep quickly but wake up too early, resulting in nighttime wakefulness and daytime sleepiness.

Many of us even think we're too busy to get a full night of what Shakespeare called that "balm of hurt minds" and "chief nourishers in life's feast."[246] Ultimately we develop what sleep experts call a "sleep debt" which we may not even know we have. According to Coren, just one hour less sleep each night for a week can cause nose dives in mood, thinking ability, attention, memory, and logical reasoning. The American Sleep

Disorder Association estimates that some 70 million Americans regularly fail to get a full night's sleep.[247] The average nightly sleep duration in America is seven and a half hours. Although about half of all older Americans say they can't get a solid night's rest, only about 20 percent of sleep disturbances are caused by underlying medical conditions.[248]

While we are asleep, the brain is busy revising and storing memory. Lack of sleep—or worse, insomnia—impairs the brain's ability to build its storehouse of information during sleep. They also result in daytime fatigue, which reduces our ability to pay attention in the first place in order to take in information accurately enough to transform it into long-term memory.

One of the ways you can help yourself get more sleep is to pick a regular bedtime (just as most of us had when we were children) and always go to bed at that same time. In the beginning you may not be sleepy, but go to bed anyway; you're programming your body to consistently relax and go to sleep. If you can't do anything else, practice your breathing. After a few days of retraining your body and mind, when you reach the bedtime you have selected, your body will be ready for sleep and you'll drop off easily.

Other ways you can help yourself get a good night's sleep include avoiding drinking alcohol and not eating heavy, hard-to-digest foods in the evening. Although alcohol is a depressant, it can disturb sleep several hours later, usually in the early morning around 2 to 3 A.M. Don't take stimulants such as tobacco (because of its nicotine) and caffeine (coffee, tea, chocolate, carbonated colas) for several hours before going to bed.

Don't exercise within two or three hours of bedtime because it can be overstimulating, causing you to have difficulty going to sleep. For a long time many experts have believed that the more active you are during the day, the less restless you will be at night and the more soundly you sleep at night. Proof that exercise during the day can help you sleep better at night was documented in a recent study done at Stanford University Medical School. Findings showed that after 16 weeks in a moderate-intensity exercise program, participants were able to fall asleep about 15 minutes earlier and sleep about 45 minutes longer at night. All the participants (29 women and 14 men) were between the ages of 50 to 74 years, lived sedentary lives, and had mild sleep complaints. They exercised at least four times a week for about 40 minutes, participating in an organized aerobics class twice a week and exercising on their own the other two days with brisk walking or stationary bike-riding.[249]

◆ **Don't Toss and Turn.** One word of warning about insomnia: if you can't manage to fall asleep after you've gone to bed and used the best relaxation techniques you know for at least half an hour, or if you wake up in the middle of the night and can't get back to sleep, don't lie there tossing and turning. You'll only succeed in getting more frustrated, and you are less likely to fall asleep. There's no point to it, you're not getting any rest. So, instead, get up and do something sedentary but pleasurable or useful. Read a good book, preferably not a thriller (because it may keep you awake), but a solid, well-written book on a subject that interests you. Or finish writing that report, which was probably causing your insomnia in the first place. Then, when you feel really sleepy, go back to bed. You'll probably fall asleep with no further problem.

Of course, you'll feel tired in the morning. But, you would have felt just as tired—and probably more tired because you would never have fallen back to sleep—if you'd stayed in bed. At least this way you've got something worthwhile to show for your tiredness. If you put up with it for the day and then go to bed at your now standardized time, you'll probably enjoy a wonderful night's sleep the following night.

Keeping Things in Perspective

A final word about stress . . .

More than any other emotion, stress is one that is within your own control. If you are sad, either in reaction to a sad event or because you are clinically depressed, there is little you can do about it by changing your attitude. The sad event remains sad. And your chemistry remains unbalanced and therefore you remain depressed until you solve the problem chemically with your doctor's help. But stress is different. It's all a matter of how you look at it. When you play a computer game, the "high" you get is very similar to the stress you feel when you are fighting traffic on your way home. But you feel totally different about the two, enjoying one experience but disliking the other. As a result, your body and your mind react differently, too.

In other words, the main difference between the two experiences is a matter of your own attitude. And that is something you *can* change. Let us give you some examples:

◆ You're late for an appointment. You could fret about it all the way there—and be ten minutes late. The people you're meeting probably won't mind; it's happened to them, too. Or you could call and say you'll be ten minutes late. You'll still get there the same ten minutes after your appointment; and the people still won't mind. But you won't be in the least stressed.

◆ You know your company is downsizing and that you're in danger of losing your job. You're worried sick; you're stressed out. Naturally, that means that you don't do your job as well. You forget more than you should. That only makes matters worse.

Instead, you take a weekend to write and hone the very best resume you can. It looks pretty solid. It's obvious you could get another job. Now when you go back to work on Monday, you feel more confident. Sure they may still fire you, but now you've started to develop your parachute. You therefore feel less stress. You forget nothing. Maybe you'll keep your job after all. Or perhaps you'll land an even better job.

You get the idea. Stress lies in the eye (or gut) of the beholder. Therefore it is within your power to change your perspective on it. Without altering the facts you can reduce the stress you feel about them. As a result, you will feel better about your life and yourself. And your memory will be considerably improved.

9

❖❖

Exercise to Maintain
Good Health

What sort of exercise?

◆

The effect of exercise on memory

❖❖

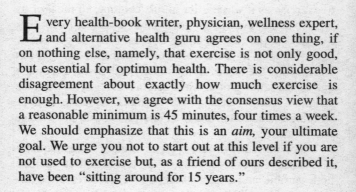

E very health-book writer, physician, wellness expert, and alternative health guru agrees on one thing, if on nothing else, namely, that exercise is not only good, but essential for optimum health. There is considerable disagreement about exactly how much exercise is enough. However, we agree with the consensus view that a reasonable minimum is 45 minutes, four times a week. We should emphasize that this is an *aim,* your ultimate goal. We urge you not to start out at this level if you are not used to exercise but, as a friend of ours described it, have been "sitting around for 15 years."

What Sort of Exercise?

The type and amount of exercise you should do, of course, depends on your age, physical condition, and your underlying health. However, here again we feel safe in recommending that, unless you have very specific health problems, you should do both aerobic and resistance exercise (i.e., lifting weights or duplicating that effort on a weight machine). The aerobic exercise is necessary to improve your cardiovascular fitness. The weight training improves the strength of both your muscles, which is important to avoid the strains and sprains of everyday living, and your bones. Yes, lifting weights actually strengthens bones, building up their mass. Thus, it counteracts and reduces the severity of osteoporosis, and greatly reduces the likelihood that you will break something. For aerobics, work out with enough vigor to keep yourself just short of breath. You should not be gasping, but you should also not be able to carry on a conversation comfortably.

Unfortunately, our current lifestyle is not as conducive to exercise as it was earlier in this century, so most of us have to make an effort to get enough exercise. According to fitness expert Dr. Kenneth Cooper, only 40 percent of adults engage in some form of moderate activity each week, while the rest of us are mostly sedentary. If you are one of the latter group, we urge you to begin an exercise program *today*. Nothing will be more effective at augmenting the action of PS or at energizing you to exercise your brain.

There are many different types of exercise, all equally satisfactory, provided you make sure that they include both aerobic and weight workouts. Therefore, the exercise you choose should largely depend on how much you enjoy it. For those people who do not enjoy any form of exercise, we sympathize but urge you to do some anyhow. The best way we know of making it at least fairly acceptable is to build as much variety into your exercise program as possible. If you dig up your garden or shovel snow (both weight exercises) one day and play squash (an aerobic exercise) another, you will be a lot less bored than pumping iron and walking on a treadmill every other day. Remember, you don't have to do both aerobics and weight-training on every occasion. As long as you do about half your total effort on each every week you will be fine.

Among the more available and pleasant exercises, we recommend:

◆ **Take More Walks.** Walking is a great, inexpensive exercise. Start out walking at a normal speed, taking about 25 or 30 minutes to walk one mile. In the next two weeks, gradually increase your speed, enabling you to walk that mile in 20 minutes. By week four you're walking one and a half miles in 30 minutes and by six weeks, you can cover two miles in less than 40 minutes. Eventually, if you have no problems with walking, by your ninth walking week you should be walking two miles in less than 35 minutes and can reduce your regimen to four times a week. If all of this seems like too much too fast, then consider it a goal to work toward, and take at least a 10- to 15-minute walk daily. As you feel more comfortable, or more daring, add 5 to 10 minutes to your walk. Gradually you will find that your energy and stamina are increasing, and you can walk longer and more rapidly.

For an interesting walk, or if it's raining, walk the local mall. Most malls encourage this and open the general area before the stores open, so people *can* walk along the corridors. Malls are heated, safe, and there are usually plenty of other walkers you can join with if you want companionship. Malls like to have walkers in the hope that they will shop after their walk. It's certainly a convenient place to have breakfast or a snack.

If you're embarrassed about exercising with others,

buy an exercise video so you can exercise in the privacy of your own home, according to your own schedule, and without commercials! Most video stores have exercise tapes for sale. If you are not motivated to exercise alone, however, you might prefer to join an exercise class. You'll find them at community centers, junior colleges, and YMCAs.

◆ **Be Sure to Warm Up and Cool Down.** Observe the rule of warming up by starting slowly and stretching for three or four minutes before exercising. Dr. Ken Cooper suggests that for older people whose bodies aren't as supple as they used to be, they should walk fairly slowly for about a quarter of a mile before stretching their Achilles tendons and hamstring muscles.[250]

When you've finished your walk, always take about five minutes to cool down by walking around at a lower, slower intensity to gradually bring your heart rate to normal. Don't lie down, sit down, or drive away. The cooldown period helps prevent the irregular heartbeat (arrhythmia) that could follow because of the enormous amounts of norepinephrine and epinephrine (blood vessel constrictor hormones) that were produced during strenuous exercise and that continue to be produced for several minutes after exercise stops.[251] This risky rhythm fluctuation reduces blood flow to the brain, and can result in dizziness. Cooling down also keeps blood from pooling in your legs. Tapering off becomes even more important as we grow older.

◆ **Consider Water Workouts.** If, because of arthritis or other disorders, you have trouble walking for exercise, don't worry. You may want to count yourself among the more than 7 million Americans who head to the swimming pool for their workout. According to the editors of the *Harvard Health Letter,* exercising in warm water can be just as effective as fast walking to stay fit and increase overall health.[252] Since many of the exercises are done in waist-deep or chest-high water, you don't have to know how to swim to get the benefits. Many YMCAs, community centers, and community colleges offer water-walking programs.

Usually water-workout group classes begin with a brief three- to five-minute warm-up, using slow movements to loosen the muscles. Then the group performs various aerobic exercises, orchestrated by an instructor, designed to raise the heart rate and work all the major muscle groups. Like land exercises, the half-hour classes end with cool-down exercises to lower the heart rate.

The United States Water Fitness Association suggests you water walk at least three times a week. To place equal emphasis on all muscles and work all muscles evenly, walk or jog an equal number of laps forward and backward. If you are not in a class, you can increase the intensity of your workout by moving your arms back and forth in and out of the water as you walk, lift your knees higher, and lift your arms higher (the higher your arms are the harder your heart will work).[253]

While strenuous exercise can temporarily increase the number of free radicals, continued training appears to augment the antioxidant defense system. Weekend athletes who do not have this augmented defense system and who may be more susceptible to tissue damage, should be sure that their antioxidant levels are adequate.

The Effect of Exercise on Memory

Exercise positively impacts memory, and slows down AAMI in two ways:

- It improves overall health, which has a generally salutary effect on all mental functions including memory.
- More specifically, it fights both stress and depression, both of which (as we explain elsewhere) interfere with memory in various ways and contribute to AAMI.

A number of studies have shown various memory-enhancing effects as a result of exercise:

- A single session of mild range-of-motion exercise in a group of cognitively unimpaired institutionalized elderly persons, aged 70+, improved recall ability for at least half an hour.[254]
- When a 12-month program of group exercise was instituted with 71 older, community-dwelling women in Australia, the exercisers showed significant improvements in reaction time, strength, memory span, and measures of well-being compared with a matched group of nonexercisers.[255]
- Another study demonstrated that exercise contributed significantly to improved moods among middle-aged and older women, regardless of whether they were premenopausal or postmenopausal, or with or without hormone replacement therapy.[256]
- The memory of 46 elderly cardiac patients with dementia and/or brain atrophy, who lived in a metropolitan city in Japan, improved significantly with exercise from walking.[257]

What all this adds up to is that exercise is good for you, your health, all your mental functions, and particularly your memory. If you are not exercising already, we urge that you start *now*.

10

When Age Isn't the Cause

Alzheimer's disease

Hypertension (high blood pressure)

Multi-infarct dementia

Alcoholism

*Wernicke-Korsakoff syndrome without
alcoholism*

Obstructive sleep apnea

Insulin dependent diabetes and hypoglycemia

Huntington's disease

Parkinson's disease

Clinical depression

Posttraumatic stress disorder

◆

Chronic fatigue syndrome

◆

The use of benzodiazepines

◆

Pregnancy

◆

Fibromyalgia

◆

Surgery

◆

Temporal lobe epilepsy

◆

Brain tumors

◆

Thyroid dysfunction

◆

Amnesia

◆

Fugue amnesia

◆

Multiple sclerosis

◆

Iron deficiency

◆

Rare diseases resulting in dementia

There are several conditions other than standard AAMI that cause us to lose our ability to learn and remember more rapidly than would normally happen with age alone. Some of those are partly curable, some are not yet. In any case, if you suspect you have any of these, you should promptly consult a physician.

Let us look now at the most frequent of these memory-harming conditions.

Alzheimer's Disease

Alzheimer's disease (AD) is a devastating, progressive, presently incurable brain disorder that, as we have mentioned previously, affects less than one out of every 20 people between 65 and 75, no more than one out of every 10 people between 75 and 85, and nearly one out of every three people over the age of 85. It is the most common cause of dementia in older people, and is believed to affect about 4 million American adults, according to the National Institute on Aging.

The disease usually begins after age 65, and the risk of acquiring it goes up with age. At present, the causes of Alzheimer's are unknown, and it is neither preventable nor curable. First-degree relatives of people with Alzheimer's disease appear to have an increased risk of developing the disorder, although definitive data are not available.[258]

We said in Chapter 1 that the cells in the body formed a complicated network. Think of it as a vast web throughout the body that communicates sensations from all over the body to that part of the web called the brain, which contains the blueprint of our cognitive abilities, our thoughts, and our memories. Destruction of brain cells, such as occurs in AD, literally wipes out the blueprint.

Result? Impaired thinking, impaired memory, and impaired behavior.

First identified in 1906 by the German physician Alois Alzheimer, in its advanced stage it progresses well beyond the normal aging process (although, as stated earlier, the early stages of AD look very much the same as AAMI). Indeed, the difference between the two is not always easy to diagnose. In fact, it took a lot of work to even lay down the definitions needed to differentiate one from the other. Before Dr. Alzheimer's discovery, the disorder was frequently described simply as "senile dementia."

In 1985, the National Institute of Mental Health (NIMH) in the United States convened a work group of experts chaired by Dr. Crook to develop criteria for operationalizing age-related memory loss that falls within the broad boundaries of normality. The group met on several occasions, and adopted the term "age-associated memory impairment," and specified a set of operational criteria for the condition. If you are in any doubt about where you stand on the AD to AAMI continuum, these criteria will help you decide for yourself. (See Table 1, page 239.)

Examination of the table reveals that the inclusion criteria are intended to select persons over 50 who are not demented, who have adequate intellectual function, who complain of gradual memory loss since early adulthood that interferes with important tasks of daily life, and who show objective evidence on performance tests that such loss has occurred. The exclusion criteria are intended to eliminate persons with any condition that might be of aetiologic significance in adult-onset memory impairment. The exclusion criteria are very similar to those employed in the diagnosis of Alzheimer's disease.[259]

TABLE 1
Age-Associated Memory Impairment:
diagnostic criteria

(1) Inclusion criteria

 (a) Males and females at least 50 years of age.

 (b) Complaints of memory loss reflected in such everyday problems as difficulty remembering names of persons after being introduced, misplacing objects, difficulty remembering telephone numbers or mailing codes, and difficulty recalling information quickly or following a distraction. Onset of memory loss must be described as gradual, without sudden worsening in recent months.

 (c) Memory test performance that is at least 1 standard deviation below the mean established for young adults on a standardized test of secondary memory (recent memory) with adequate normative data. Examples of specific tests and appropriate cutoff scores follow, although other measures of adequate normative data are equally appropriate:

 Benton Visual Retention Test (Benton, 1963) (number correct, Administration A)   7 or less

 Logical memory subtest of the Wechsler Memory Scale (WMS) (Weschler and Stone, 1983)   6 or less

 Associate Learning subtest of the WMS (score on "hard" associates)   6 or less

 (d) Evidence of adequate intellectual function as determined by a scaled score of at least 9 (raw score of at least 32) on the Vocabulary Subtest of the Wechsler Adult Intelligence Scale (Wechsler, 1955).

 (e) Absence of dementia as determined by a score of 24 or higher on the Mini-Mental State Examination (Folstein et al., 1975). Many investigators have chosen a score of 27 rather than 24 to exclude questionable cases of dementia.

(2) Exclusion criteria

 (a) Evidence of delirium, confusion, or other disturbances of consciousness.

(b) Any neurologic disorder that could produce cognitive deterioration as determined by history, clinical neurologic examination, and, if indicated, neuroradiologic examination. Such disorders include AD, Parkinson's disease, stroke, intracranial hemorrhage, local brain lesions, including tumors, and normal pressure hydrocephalus.

(c) History of any infective or inflammatory brain disease, including viral, fungal, and syphilitic.

(d) Evidence of significant cerebral vascular disease as determined by a Hachinski Ischaemia Score (modified version: Rosen et al., 1980) of 4 or more or by neuroradiologic examination.

(e) History of repeated minor head injury (as in boxing) or single injury resulting in a period of unconsciousness for 1 hour or more.

(f) Current psychiatric diagnosis according to DSM-IIIR (American Psychological Association, 1980) criteria of depression, mania, or any major psychiatric disorder.

(g) Current diagnosis or history of alcoholism or drug dependence.

(h) Evidence of depression as determined by a Hamilton Depression Rating Scale (Hamilton, 1967) score of 13 or more.

(i) Any medical disorder that could produce cognitive deterioration, including renal, respiratory, cardiac, and hepatic disease; diabetes melitis unless well controlled by diet or oral hypoglycaemic agents; endocrine, metabolic, or hematologic disturbances; and malignancy not in remission for more than 2 years. Determination should be based on complete medical history, clinical examination (including electrocardiogram), and appropriate laboratory tests.

(j) Use of any psychotropic drug or any other drug that may significantly affect cognitive function during the month before psychometric testing.

Since 1985, various modifications have been made to these original criteria, but no fundamental changes have occurred. Thus, the above definitions are effectively still the way we differentiate AD from AAMI.

Even though the small group of pioneers who conducted research on the disease in the 1970s has expanded to thousands of scientists all over the world, the cause of AD is still unknown. The means by which brain cells in AD die much more rapidly than in AAMI is a matter of intensive study. Much of the evidence points to a factor known as *beta-amyloid protein,* which is a major component in the nerve cells. Although beta-amyloid, a waxy substance consisting of some protein combined with certain carbohydrates, is present in normal brains and has a normal biological function, the brains of AD patients seem to produce an overabundance. This very high concentration is toxic to nerve cells[260] and may cause the hippocampal neurons to degenerate, so that short-term memory and the ability to perform routine tasks begin to falter. As the disease spreads through the cerebral cortex, it begins to take away language. In its final stages, the disease wipes out a person's ability to recognize even close family members or to communicate in any way, leaving them completely dependent on others for care.

Researchers have found some genetic abnormalities on chromosome 21 in persons with early-onset AD, which is quite rare and typically occurs between the ages of 40 and 50. They are not sure about the genetic component of cases of the disease that occur at more advanced ages, but, certainly, scientists the world over have kicked into high gear the search for other flaws in the genetic code. They have now discovered genetic abnormalities in two additional chromosomes, 1 and 14, in families where AD follows a certain inheritance pattern.

A current theory regarding AD is that it may not be one disease but several. Possible causes that researchers are investigating include a slow virus, environmental toxins, and chemical imbalance in the brain. Research points to AD probably not being caused by any one facto rather by several risk factors that combine or act differently in each person.

In AD, nerve-cell death begins insidiously, many years before the onset of memory loss or any other symptoms. During that time, remaining nerve cells compensate, and it is only when the last remaining cells in a particular area of the brain die that symptoms begin.

The groundbreaking Nun Study—involving more than 100 nuns of the School Sisters of Notre Dame religious order in Mankato, Minnesota—included an examination of the brains of 14 of the nuns who had died (ages 75 to 95 years), 10 of whom had Alzheimer's. The study hints that the subtle beginnings of Alzheimer's could actually be present *up to 60 years* before it is recognized, perhaps even while future sufferers are quite young. Among the 14 nuns who died, autopsies confirmed that all those with Alzheimer's disease had relatively poor language skills ("low idea density") in their early twenties, as determined by autobiographies written at that time. None of the deceased sisters with high idea density had Alzheimer's.[261] Although the study indicates that low linguistic ability in early life may be a strong predictor of poor cognitive function and AD in late life, for the nuns, like most people, symptoms are not obvious until much later in life.

As stated, the actual diagnosis of probable Alzheimer's is only possible through cognitive tests with the definitive examination for the hallmark traits of the disease only identifiable by autopsy. Even then, if the patient is over 75 years old, pathologists often disagree ... as noted earlier, the same structural brain ... at occur in AD also occur in AAMI. The ob... largely quantitative, and experts disagree on ... of neurofibrilly tangles and plaques constitute AD. Nevertheless, the cognitive diagnoses are reasonably accurate. When the brains of 2,200 people who had sought evaluation for signs of dementia before death were examined in autopsy, the 200 people diagnosed cognitively with probable AD before death were actually found to have some other form of dementia.[262]

After diagnosis, the average survival of people with AD ranges from four to eight years, although some may live for as long as 20 years. Typically they die from pneumonia or other diseases and AD is not reported on the death certificate.

The drug Aricept may slightly alleviate some cognitive symptoms, and other medications may be of substantial help in controlling such behavioral symptoms of AD as sleeplessness, agitation, wandering, anxiety, and depression. Treating these symptoms often helps Alzheimer's patients be more comfortable and makes their care a little easier for caregivers. However, sadly, nothing close to a cure is yet available.

Since many conditions that result in severe memory loss or dementia—such as vitamin deficiency, thyroid disease, certain infections, drug reactions, circulatory disease, brain tumors, small brain infarcts, head injuries, and depression—are arrestable, reversible, or even preventable, a complete medical and neurological evaluation is vital whenever an individual begins to experience significant memory problems.

Hypertension (High Blood Pressure)

A number of researchers are now assessing the relationship between blood pressure and intellectual function in both laboratory animals and older humans. Like advanced age, essential hypertension, a chronic disorder, has been associated with changes in brain morphology and cognitive function. Long-standing untreated hypertension causes reductions in cerebral blood flow, oxygen metabolism, and vascular lesions in the brain's white matter, all leading to impaired cognitive functioning.[263] In general, scientists have found that humans with hypertension perform more poorly than those with normal blood pressure (called "normotensives") on tests of memory, attention, and abstract reasoning.[264]

Studies in both Brazil and Mexico have determined that when aging rats that have spontaneously developed hypertension are compared with rats that have not, their training and subsequent performance in learning and running mazes showed a decrease in learning, memory, and spontaneous activity.[265] Researchers at the University of Alabama showed, however, that they could prevent the decline in learning and memory skills by giving the rats captopril, an antihypertensive drug.[266]

Researchers continue to try to answer the question of whether drug therapy for hypertension worsens, improves, or leaves unaltered objectively measured cognitive skills. Back in the second half of the 1960s, a landmark long-term study, then known as the Honolulu Heart Program, was begun. It measured, among a number of other things, the blood pressure of the Japanese-American men living in Hawaii who participated in the study. In the years 1991 through 1993, 3,735 men (average age 78 years) were reexamined for a fourth time. Results showed that the level of systolic blood pressure (the first number in a blood pressure reading) in midlife was a significant predictor of reduced cognitive function in later life, suggesting that early control of systolic pressure may reduce the risk of cognitive impairment in old age. The level of cognitive function was not associated with midlife diastolic blood pressure (the second number in the reading).[267]

A study conducted at Hammersmith Hospital in London compared 69 people (ages 70 to 84 years) who were diagnosed as hypertensive and had not previously received antihypertensive treatment with captopril or bendrofluazide. Those whose diastolic blood pressure was lowered the most improved their cognitive scores (sentence repetition and recall of paired words) compared to those who were the least responsive to the medication. This study, at least, suggests that long-term adequate blood pressure control may reverse some of the cognitive impairment associated with preexisting hypertension.[268]

Finnish researchers discovered that the performance on a series of tests to evaluate cognitive function involving calculation and semantic memory was definitely impaired for a group of 378 hypertensive people compared to the performance of a normotensive group of 366 persons. Although all the participants were nondiabetic, those persons with hypertension who also had a high insulin level after fasting scored even worse in 16 of the 19 tests that measured calculation, language, semantic memory, and problem-solving than did hypertensive subjects with normal insulin levels.[269]

When researchers at the Laboratory of Neurosciences at the National Institute on Aging in Bethesda, Maryland, compared "young-old" people (ages 56 to 69) with hypertension and "old-old" (ages 70–84) hypertensive people with age-matched people without hypertension, they found that hypertension exacerbates structural changes in the brain accompanying advanced age. Not only did researchers use magnetic resonance imaging (MRI) of the brain to measure the size of different brain structures and the volume of cerebrospinal fluid, they also administered a battery of neuropsychological tests to each person. The combined hypertensive groups showed poorer performance in memory and language tests.[270]

A study which tested 1,695 stroke-free participants in the Framingham Heart Study suggests, however, that the odds of performing poorly on certain visual and verbal neuropsychological tests were higher for age than for blood pressure, although blood pressure and chronic hypertension also resulted in poor performance.[271] Thus, age has a much stronger association with memory loss than does blood pressure, but there is a high probability that hypertension, particularly in later life, can contribute to declines in memory and other cognitive abilities.

In 1995, doctors at Duke looked at the possibility that there was a genetic link to impaired cognitive abilities in people with hypertension, and found that it was likely. Sixty-two hypertensive men and women who reported a family history of hypertension were compared with 28 hypertensive individuals without such a family history and 32 normotensive controls. Each person individually took a battery of tests that included information processing, and verbal and figural memory. Results showed that those people with a family history did poorer on tests of attention and short-term memory than people in either of the other two groups, although there were no differences between the groups on tests of verbal or figural memory.[272]

Multi-Infarct Dementia

When brain damage occurs because of a series of successive small strokes, it is called *multi-infarct dementia* (infarct means the closing of a blood vessel). These small strokes, or what are called "cerebrovascular accidents," cause brief periods of "spacing out" that typically last less than a minute. They are caused when the blood supply to an area of the brain becomes blocked, gradually destroying brain tissue. Often they are associated with high blood pressure or diabetes, both of which damage blood vessels in the brain.[273]

About 20 percent of all cases of severe cognitive dysfunction and dementia in the elderly are due to such a series of small strokes. In fact overall, multi-infarct dementia is the second most common cause of dementia.[274] Unlike AD, where the symptoms develop slowly over time, symptoms of multi-infarct dementia can occur quite suddenly. Nevertheless, the cognitive deficits seen in the two conditions are often quite similar.

Alcoholism

In a study conducted at the Health Science Center in Brooklyn, New York, not surprisingly, 77 alcoholics did worse on a test of short-term memory than did 48 nonalcoholic controls. The alcoholics demonstrated more errors and longer response time. Electrophysiological information suggested that long-term alcohol abuse results in deficits in information encoding and hence difficulty in remembering the information.[275]

When a study was done on alcohol consumption and cognitive functioning on 2,040 randomly selected African-Americans, it was found that subjects in the heaviest drinking category (more than 20 drinks per week) scored the poorest in cognitive tests and scales of daily functioning. Surprisingly, the scores of lifetime abstainers were worse than those of people in the lightest drinking category (fewer than four drinks per week). The differences between the drinking categories were modest, however, and the clinical significance of the study remains uncertain until further studies are conducted.[276]

While alcoholism typically leads to only mild memory impairment, some of the most striking cases of memory loss or amnesia result from a condition, *Korsakoff's syndrome,* which afflicts chronic alcoholics who have eaten a poor diet and have developed thiamine (Vitamin B_{12}) deficiency. A person with Korsakoff's syndrome loses their memory of recent events, and may make up stories to try to cover the inability to remember. They are "stuck" in the past and unable to remember later portions of their life. They may also show little affect. The condition is named for the nineteenth-century Russian psychiatrist Sergei Korsakoff, who first described it. Korsakoff's syndrome sometimes follows a bout of delirium tremens, and the disorder can be fatal unless the thiamine deficiency is treated.[277]

In some people, *Wernicke's encephalopathy* is a precursor to Korsakoff's syndrome. They suddenly become disoriented and confused. They have abnormal eye movements, other uncoordinated movements, and abnormal nerve function. Memory and accompanying emotional behavior may change dramatically from one moment to the next. When this confusional state ends, people who have not received immediate treatment emerge with the chronic and debilitating memory impairment of Korsakoff's amnesia.[278]

Chronic alcoholism can also damage or destroy the myelin sheath, the insulation wrapped around nerve fibers, causing nerve damage, which may be minimal if the sheath is able to repair and regenerate itself, or irreversible if the destruction is extensive. Such damage will typically destroy a good deal of memory capacity.

Wernicke-Korsakoff Syndrome Without Alcoholism

Researchers have concluded that what were once considered two separate syndromes, Korsakoff's and Wernicke's, are in fact one. Korsakoff's syndrome emphasized the mental symptoms, while Wernicke's emphasized the neurological symptoms, but they are both aspects of the same condition. Wernicke-Korsakoff syndrome is caused not only by alcoholism, but also by infection, cerebral hemorrhage, and postsurgical complications. Consuming large quantities of refined sugars can result in thiamine deficiency, which can lead to the syndrome. Symptoms tend to reappear when stress is placed on the person. Drs. Abram Hoffer and Morton Walker, authors of *Smart Nutrients,* think it is possible that many senile people are examples of Wernicke-Korsakoff syndrome where initial stresses of age have precipitated another outburst of symptoms or there is a long-standing thiamine deficiency.[279]

Obstructive Sleep Apnea

The chronic sleep disruption that results from obstructive sleep apnea (OSA) can also adversely affect memory. The fundamental problem in OSA is the periodic collapse or relaxation of the pharyngeal airway during sleep. Airflow is impeded by the collapsed pharynx, choking off respiration, which increasingly stimulates breathing efforts against the collapsed airway, typically until the person is awakened after about 10 seconds of oxygen deprivation.[280] Males are eight times more commonly affected than females, although after menopause the gap narrows considerably. Sleep apnea can occur in children, usually in relation to large tonsils and adenoids, but in adult life it usually occurs between the ages of 40 and 60, and the prevalence increases with age.[281] Apnea is especially common among individuals who are overweight, because fat in the neck area puts extra pressure on breathing passages.

It is common for people with sleep apnea to have excessive daytime sleepiness. As the disorder progresses, that sleepiness becomes increasingly "irresistible" and dangerous, and patients develop cognitive dysfunction, inability to concentrate, memory and judgment impairment, irritability, and depression, say researchers at the Medical School of Pennsylvania State University.[282]

When French scientists at the National Institute of Health and Medical Research in Paris evaluated 1,389 men and women living in Nantes in western France, those who self-reported breathing stoppage during sleep (10.8 percent), or that had been told that they snore (49.5 percent), scored poorest on several of the cognitive tests. The relationships were significant only when either snoring or apnea was also associated with daytime sleepiness.[283] Apparently, poor cognitive functioning during the day goes hand-in-hand with daytime sleepiness.

Researchers in the Department of Psychology at the University of Kentucky compared eight elderly patients diagnosed with sleep apnea with 12 healthy controls, and found that those with sleep apnea were more depressed and had lower scores on various memory tests.[284]

Insulin Dependent Diabetes and Hypoglycemia

Severe hypoglycemia (low blood sugar) is known to have deleterious effects on the hippocampus, and research indicates that even a modest increase in circulating glucose levels enhances memory. Laboratory studies with rats suggest that glucose (sugar) may enhance memory by increasing the release of acetylcholine.[285] The body first responds to a drop in blood sugar by releasing epinephrine from the adrenal glands. This, in turn, stimulates the release of sugar from body stores, causing symptoms similar to those of an anxiety attack: sweating, nervousness, and confusion. More severe hypoglycemia reduces the glucose supply to the brain, causing dizziness, headache, inability to concentrate, and difficulty in organizing memories coherently. Prolonged hypoglycemia may permanently damage the brain.[286]

Huntington's Disease

Huntington's disease is a devastating hereditary illness that eventually destroys the brain's motor system, which carries a form of procedural memory. The symptoms that stem from damage to the basal ganglia, a subcortical collection of structures, can start at any age, but in most cases begin between ages 30 and 50.

Parkinson's Disease

Parkinson's disease is a slowly progressing disorder that results when nerve cells in the basal ganglia degenerate. The basal ganglia process signals and transmits messages to the thalamus. Their main neurotransmitter is dopamine, and their steady degeneration results in a lower production of dopamine and fewer connections with other nerve cells and muscles.

The major cause of deterioration is unknown, but occasionally it is one of the late complications of viral encephalitis. Any drug or toxin that interferes with the production or action of dopamine, such as antipsychotic drugs used to treat severe paranoia and schizophrenia, can also cause irreversible symptoms of Parkinson's disease.[287]

Often, the disease begins with a tremor in the hand, although not always. About a third of the patients with Parkinson's develop some symptoms of dementia, but most people maintain normal intellect. Memory impairment, however, especially explicit memory (verbal recall of words and drawings), occurs in most patients. Some aspects of memory[288] are affected as well.

Clinical Depression

While nearly everyone may occasionally have "the blues" or a "down" day, about 15 percent of all adults experience at least one episode of serious or disabling depression at some time in their lives. Incidents of depression appear to be on the rise, since visits to doctors for depression doubled between the last half of the 1980s and the first half of the 1990s. According to the American Psychiatric Association, 11 million people visited doctors for depression in 1988, a number that increased to over 20 million in 1993–94.[289]

In addition to profound sadness or complete loss of interest in everyday activities, other symptoms of depression include loss of appetite, insomnia, restlessness, persistent fatigue, feelings of inadequacy, difficulty making decisions, and thoughts about death or suicide. It is also well known that people experiencing clinical depression can experience memory loss, especially with regard to short-term memory. Ten women ranging in age from 70 to 81 years who were hospitalized for depression were treated with a placebo for 15 days, followed by 300 milligrams daily of PS for 30 days. Depressive symptoms did not change after administration of the placebo, but were significantly reduced with the PS therapy. While PS is not specifically an antidepressant, it is important to note that consistent improvements occurred in recall and long-term memory.[290]

The reasons that depression causes memory loss are not completely clear. Perhaps the noticeable memory reduction is not a fundamental breakdown in the process of memorization due to depression, but merely the result of the lowered motivation experienced during depression.[291] When you are depressed, remembering certain kinds of new information simply does not seem important.

Reactive depression, such as that which often occurs with grief, in response to death of a person or beloved pet, or any significant loss or change (moving, retirement, long-lasting physical impairment), decreases your ability to concentrate on outside matters and, therefore, also can impair your memory. This type of memory problem usually lessens over time as the process of mourning progresses and the mourner gradually recovers.

The reduction in the quantity or conductivity of certain neurotransmitters, like serotonin and norepinephrine, that are related to memory may also contribute to the combination of loss of memory and depression. Hormonal changes associated with the menses, pregnancy, childbirth, and menopause can also contribute to depression.

Posttraumatic Stress Disorder

Posttraumatic stress disorder (PTSD) is an anxiety condition caused by exposure to an overwhelming traumatic event. At some time in the future, and with some regularity, the person reexperiences the event in nightmares or flashbacks. Sometimes symptoms don't begin until months or even years after the event. Common symptoms include a numbing of general responsiveness, difficulty falling asleep, being easily startled, and depression. PTSD slowly becomes less intense over time, even without treatment, although some people remain severely handicapped indefinitely. Treatment of PTSD involves behavior therapy, antidepressant and antianxiety drugs, and psychotherapy.[292]

When veterans of the Persian Gulf War were studied, those with PTSD showed deficiencies on tasks of sustained attention, mental manipulation, initial acquisition of information, and retroactive interference. Some models of PTSD suggest that the memory difficulties experienced by people suffering from PTSD are related to hyperarousal and dysfunction of the frontal-subcortical systems,[293] which may be the result of stress-induced alterations.[294]

Over time, many studies have documented the memory deficits among combat veterans with PTSD; however, high rates of post-combat anxiety, depression, alcoholism, and substance abuse have often made it difficult to establish PTSD as the main culprit in memory loss. To compensate for this, researchers in San Diego examined the learning and memory functioning of rape survivors without alcoholism or substance abuse but with PTSD and compared it to the cognitive functions of rape victims without PTSD. Those with PTSD performed significantly worse on tasks of delayed free recall, strengthening the theory that memory deficits are associated with PTSD.[295]

Chronic Fatigue Syndrome

As its name implies, chronic fatigue syndrome (CFS) is an illness that is characterized by severe and prolonged fatigue that affects both physical and mental functioning. Other symptoms include impaired concentration and memory, disturbed sleep, depressed mood, and anxiety.[296] In some cases these symptoms are accompanied by a low-grade fever and swelling of the lymph nodes.[297]

Controversy has raged as to CFS's etiology, with suggestions ranging from various physical and psychosocial stressors, to viruses, to psychiatric disturbances rather than physical measures being more predictive of long-term disability.[298] A number of researchers have noted that there is a disparity between the degree of CFS patients' complaints about the actual degree of impairment, and researchers in Great Britain have found that severity of complaints about failing memory was more related to accompanying depression than to CFS. On balance, CFS appears to reduce memory to some extent in its sufferers, largely middle-aged, upper social-level females. However, there is little known about its causes or solutions.

The Use of Benzodiazepines

We mentioned earlier that certain medications can result in memory impairment. Benzodiazepines, such as the tranquilizers Librium, Valium, and Halcion, used to treat psychological symptoms such as anxiety and sleep disorders are particularly likely to cause these symptoms. Benzodiazepines promote mental and physical relaxation by reducing nerve activity in the brain; hence, they can also impair memory, result in memory loss and diminished attention span, and may even cause a person to appear to have dementia, i.e., to speak slowly and have difficulty in thinking and understanding others. After benzodiazepines were discovered, they replaced barbiturates as the drug of choice for the treatment of anxiety.

Although safer than barbiturates, they are, nevertheless, addictive if taken over a long time and must be tapered off slowly rather than stopped abruptly, because withdrawal can produce potentially life-threatening reactions similar to those experienced in alcohol withdrawal. The elderly, who can't metabolize and excrete drugs as well as younger people, may be particularly susceptible to the memory impairment effects of benzodiazepines.[299] When the functional status of a group of 4,192 adults 65 years of age and older was determined by their reports of their activities of daily living, those exposed to a benzodiazepine during the previous 12 months had a lower functional status. The use of benzodiazepines impaired functional status as much as some chronic medical conditions.[300]

Pregnancy

Many women believe that pregnancy impairs their memory. When 48 volunteer pregnant women were compared with 19 nonpregnant controls, 39 (81 percent) of the pregnant women rated their memory as being impaired, while only 3 (16 percent) of the nonpregnant women did. Objective tests of recall, recognition, and priming memory (where some memory of a recent event remains in the brain, even when a person is unaware of it) showed that the pregnant women were significantly impaired in the recall of both lists of words and priming memory. No conclusions have been reached about the cause of the impaired memory.[301]

Fibromyalgia

Fibromyalgia is a rheumatic disorder characterized by the presence of widespread musculoskeletal pain and tender points on the body. Muscle tightness and spasms may also occur. The pain and stiffness may occur throughout the body or may be restricted to certain locations. Fibromyalgia throughout the body is more common in women, while men are more likely to develop it in a particular area. Other symptoms include sleep disturbance, fatigue, anxiety, depression, and irritable bowel syndrome.[302] One of the most prominent complaints of patients with fibromyalgia is impaired cognitive ability including reduced memory.

At the University of Michigan, new research is being conducted to investigate the cognitive and neuroendocrine functions of patients with fibromyalgia, the theory being that patients with fibromyalgia may have both cognitive and neuroendocrine functions similar to that of control subjects who are 20 to 30 years older.[303] If so, the development of fibromyalgia may teach us something about memory in relation to aging.

Surgery

Fuzzy thinking, or a sense that their memory just wasn't the same, is a complaint that surgeons often hear from their patients after surgery. Now there is some validation for these complaints. Researchers from seven European countries and the United States tested more than 1,200 people, aged 60 or older, before major noncardic surgery that would require general anesthesia, and then retested them one week after surgery. In 26 percent of the cases there was cognitive dysfunction, i.e., confusion, memory loss, or concentration problems. At three months after surgery, mental function was still impaired in 10 percent of the participants. Although confusion and memory loss in the first few days after surgery may be expected due to the lingering effects of drugs used for anesthesia or pain control, age seems a major factor in changes that last longer. People between the ages of 70 and 80 were twice as likely to have long-term mental impairment as people between the ages of 60 and 70.[304]

Temporal Lobe Epilepsy

Epilepsy is a broad term for a variety of brain disorders characterized by the tendency to have recurring seizures, which may be triggered by a number of different things, such as repetitive sounds and flashing lights. Brain scans (MRI imaging) in people with epilepsy may uncover microscopic scarring, possibly due to brain injury at birth, or an electroencephalogram (EEG) may reveal abnormal electrical activity (alterations in brain wave patterns). Some people develop epilepsy following surgery or some type of injury to the brain, as from a stroke, a tumor, or an accident. A few types of juvenile epilepsy are thought to be inherited. Seizures can usually be prevented with medication, but that may cause drowsiness, sedation, or memory impairments.

The temporal lobes, which are involved in comprehending sounds and images, play a large part in processing immediate events into recent and long-term memory. An injury to the right temporal lobe can result in right temporal lobe epilepsy. This tends to impair memory of sounds and shapes. Damage to the left temporal lobe (left temporal lobe epilepsy) interferes with the understanding of language and may prevent people from expressing themselves or being able to cluster information appropriately. Consequently, their memory of facts and events may be impaired.[305]

Brain Tumors

Last year, some 100,000 Americans were diagnosed with brain tumors, almost double the number of a decade ago.[306] A tumor is an abnormal mass anywhere in the body and can be malignant (cancerous) or benign (non-cancerous), but either way an abnormal growth in the brain can cause considerable damage, perhaps more so than in other areas of the body.

Although refinements in surgical tools have made tumor removal more precise and safe, benign tumors that lie deep within the brain often cannot be removed because of resulting damage to other parts of the brain. As the mass grows, it can damage areas that are even far from the tumor, and as it presses on surrounding tissue, it can become life-threatening.

There are a number of different types of brain tumors, and the symptoms depend on their size, growth rate, and location. Meningiomas or benign tumors that originate in the meninges or covering around the brain can cause memory loss and difficulty in thinking. Some tumors can cause seizures; others can affect our sight, hearing, and sense of smell.[307]

Thyroid Dysfunction

The thyroid is a small gland that lies just under the skin below the Adam's apple in the neck. Normally the gland can't be seen and can barely be felt. It secretes thyroid hormones that control the body's metabolic rate (the speed at which chemical functions proceed). A number of disorders can result when thyroid functioning goes awry. Most common are *hyperthyroidism,* which results when the gland is overactive and produces too much hormone, and *hypothyroidism,* when too little hormone is produced.[308]

In hyperthyroidism, the body's functions speed up and older people can become confused. In hypothyroidism, older people sometimes become weak, sleepy, withdrawn, and depressed. In either case, their memories may decline.

A number of studies with laboratory animals have shown that manipulation of various hormones, such as thyroid, gonadal, and adrenal hormones, change the physiological development of the hippocampus, thereby affecting learning and memory.[309] Hyperthyroidism in rats significantly impaired spatial learning ability.[310]

Hypothyroidism develops when the thyroid gland is underactive and causes bodily functions to slow down. The symptoms are subtle and gradual and may be mistaken for depression. Older people especially may appear confused, forgetful, or demented, signs that may be mistaken for Alzheimer's disease or other forms of dementia.[311] Very severe hypothyroidism is called myxedema, and studies indicate that memory loss in myxedematous patients ranges between 23 to 55 percent.[312]

At the Jewish Homes for the Aging in Reseda, California, researchers were able to associate hypothyroidism in nondemented older adults with various learning and memory impairments (word fluency, visual-spatial abilities, and some aspects of attention, visual scanning, and motor speed.)[313]

Researchers in Italy were among the first to recognize that even subclinical hypothyroidism (a borderline condition of inadequate thyroid functioning) is associated with memory impairment, which can be improved by treatment with levothyroxine,[314] or L-thyroxine.[315] Middle-age and older patients in Ontario, Canada, were diagnosed with subclinical hypothyroidism because, although they showed none of the symptoms associated with hypothyroidism, they had elevated levels of thyroid-stimulating hormone (TSH) in their blood. When treated with thyroxine, their memory improved significantly more than that of nontreated or control patients.[316]

Amnesia

Simply defined, amnesia is the inability to remember past experiences. Most of us have amnesia of our infancy. One theory suggests that, because the myelin that is needed to wrap and insulate axons has not yet developed, the ability to retain messages in sequence is impaired. Other more psychologically oriented theorists hold that it has little or nothing to do with specialized neurological development, but rather that our autobiographical memory only emerges contemporaneously with the "cognitive self," a "knowledge structure" that allows us to organize memories of experiences that happened to "me." Because this cognitive self emerges in the second year of life, the lower limit for early autobiographical memories is set at about that age.[317] We don't see why one theory necessarily precludes the other. Possibly they are both correct.

Loss of memory that occurs as a result of some trauma or injury to the brain, such as might occur in an accident with a resulting concussion, or with a brain tumor, is also referred to as amnesia. *Retrograde amnesia* refers to the ability to remember things that occur after the trauma, but forgetting facts from months or even years before the occurrence. Another type, *anterograde amnesia,* occurs when the events before the trauma may be remembered, but facts following it will not be. This results in an inability to learn new facts or skills and may reflect an underlying limbic or neurochemical dysfunction.[318]

A third type of amnesia, *global transitory amnesia,* refers to the kind of memory loss that lasts a short time and may involve facts both before and after the event. It is frequently caused by a temporary decrease of blood flow to the brain (doctors call it *cerebral ischemia*), usually from some sudden trauma. You may recall that, for quite some time after the automobile accident that killed Princess Diana, her driver could not remember what happened at the time of the accident, but gradually his memory returned. Sometimes a brief residue of information acquired shortly before the trauma never comes back. With repeated head injury, such as that which occurs in boxers, progressive memory loss and cognitive functioning can develop even after boxing has been abandoned.

Fugue Amnesia

From time to time a person's life becomes so extreme or stressful that the desire to escape it is preeminent. When that happens, he or she may "blank out" for a few weeks or months. Also called functional, hysterical, and psychogenic amnesia, it is relatively rare even though it frequently and dramatically occurs in fictional television shows and in movies, where a dramatic blow to the head

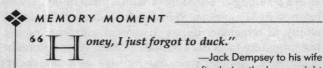

❖ MEMORY MOMENT _____

"**H**oney, I just forgot to duck."

—Jack Dempsey to his wife
after losing the heavyweight
title to Gene Tunney
on September 23, 1926.

causes the amnesia, and the plot is resolved when another blow to the head restores memory and . . . "they live happily ever after." In truth, although a blow to the head can cause some amnesias, a second blow to the head is likely to simply cause more damage.

People suffering from this type of memory loss are generally oblivious to their disconnection from the past until a situation arises that requires them to provide information about their identity or background.[319]

One expert suggests that psychogenic amnesia is actually the failure to properly understand information initially, thus obviously making it harder or impossible to retrieve.[320] Other experts believe that one of the major characteristics of functional amnesia is a process called *dissociation*, where memory systems that ordinarily communicate in some way "lose touch with each other" so that large portions of experience are no longer available to a person's conscious awareness. Dissociation also plays a major role in cases of multiple personality disorder (MPD). Now officially re-termed *dissociative identity disorder*, MPD is also a very rare disorder in spite of the almost mass emergence in the past 10 years of people claiming to have it.

Multiple Sclerosis

In this degenerative disorder, the nerves of the eye, brain, and spinal cord lose multiple patches of the myelin sheath. When myelin is damaged, nerves can't conduct impulses properly, so symptoms depend on the area affected. The cause of multiple sclerosis (MS) is unknown, but some experts believe that a virus or some unknown antigen somehow triggers an autoimmune process, causing the body to produce antibodies against its own myelin. The antibodies provoke inflammation and damage the myelin sheath. Heredity plays a small role in multiple sclerosis, as does environment. About 5 percent of people with the disease have a sibling who is also affected, and about 15 percent have a close relative. The climate in which a person spends the first decade of life also appears to play some role. One out of every 2,000 people who spent it in a temperate climate develop multiple sclerosis, whereas it afflicts only one out of every 10,000 people who spend their first decade in a tropical climate.[321]

Studies have consistently found that multiple sclerosis patients perform poorly on tests of long-term memory, but it is unclear how remote events or autobiographical memories are affected. In two studies by Dr. William Beatty and colleagues, MS patients were found to be significantly impaired on tests that required the identification of pictures of famous people and recall of public events from the 1940s to the 1970s. The results were not linked to visual impairments.[322] A larger study, however, required participants to recall the last eight U.S. presidents in chronological order, and although MS patients recalled fewer presidents than normal controls, the difference was not statistically significant.[323]

To clarify this issue, one of Dr. Beatty's students, Robert H. Paul, and other colleagues at the University of Oklahoma, used an autobiographical memory interview (AMI) with 44 MS patients and 19 normal controls matched for age, education, and gender. Autobiographical memory, one measure of remote memory, had never been tested in MS until this study. The AMI requires respondents to recall both semantic and episodic memories from three life periods: childhood, early adult, and recent adult. The investigators also used a shortened version of the "famous faces" test (15 pictures from the

1980s and 10 pictures from the 1990s), the test of recall of past U.S. presidents (the last eight presidents of the U.S. in reverse order beginning with the president currently in office), and a 14-word learning list. MS patients performed significantly lower on the learning list and the famous faces test, but not on recall of past presidents.[324]

Iron Deficiency

Iron deficiency, even when so mild as not to cause amnesia, can interfere with learning and memory, especially in adolescent girls who are prone to iron deficiency owing to poor appetite, skipping meals, and menstrual bleeding. In a study of 78 adolescent girls with nonanemic iron deficiency, pediatricians at Johns Hopkins University School of Medicine treated half of them with 650 milligrams twice daily of ferrous sulphate pills. The other girls received a placebo.[325]

Before and after treatment, all underwent four tests of attention and memory to measure cognitive functioning, including their ability to recall a list of 12 newly learned words. After eight weeks of treatment, those girls who had received iron were able to recall significantly more words, while the placebo group did not improve.

For those of us who are adults, however, we may have enough, or even too much iron. In 1992, an intriguing study conducted on 2,000 middle-aged men in eastern Finland, found that every 1 percent increase in a man's level of iron increased his risk of heart attack by 4 percent.

So, while we don't suggest that you cut back on iron, we do suggest if you have been feeling weak, fatigued, with achy joints, decreased stamina, and a decreased sexual desire (all symptoms of iron deficiency), that you have tests to see whether or not you actually need more iron.[326]

Cooked oysters are one of the best iron-containing foods. Other foods that contain iron include beef, poultry, and fish, some vegetables (lima beans, broccoli, potatoes, peas), and raisins. Eating other foods that contain Vitamin C allows the body to hold onto a greater amount of the iron in other foods, while coffee and tea taken with food can decrease iron absorption.

Rare Diseases Resulting in Dementia

A rare degenerative dementia, *Pick's disease* is named after the Prague psychiatrist, Arnold Pick, who discovered it. Behavior often appears similar to that of people with AD, but it may develop more slowly. Resulting from an atrophy in the frontal and/or temporal areas, as revealed by a CAT scan, Pick's disease is characterized by a progressive degeneration of mental faculties, especially the increasing failure to understand language or to express one's ideas (called *aphasia*).

A relatively rare progressive disease caused by an infection of the brain, *Creutzfeldt-Jakob disease* is distinguished from other forms of dementia by the rapid deterioration of mental faculties, accompanied by muscle twitching. The disease primarily affects adults, particularly those in their late fifties. It is transmissible from tissue to tissue, and a few people have acquired it from receiving contaminated corneal or other tissue transplants from infected donors or from contaminated instruments used during brain surgery. The causative organism has been difficult to identify but is suspected to be a specific protein called a *prion*. For months or years after exposure no symptoms occur. Slowly, brain damage and the accompanying loss of intellectual ability increases in the always fatal disease. Then suddenly the symptoms of the fatal disease accelerate much more rapidly than with Alzheimer's disease.[327] This is the disease which caused the death of George Balanchine, the noted director of the New York City Ballet.

Wilson's disease is a rare (affects 1 out of 30,000 people) hereditary disorder in which copper accumulation in the tissues of the body causes extensive damage. Because the liver fails to secrete copper into the blood or excrete copper into the bile, the copper level in the blood is low, but copper accumulates in the brain, eyes, and liver (causing cirrhosis). The accumulated copper produces golden brown or gray-green rings (called the *Kayser-Fleischer ring*) in the cornea of the eyes. When the copper accumulation in the brain is sufficient to destroy the nerve cells, neurologic symptoms begin, the most common of which include tremor of the extremities, lack of coordination, headaches, and dementia with accompanying personality changes.

The untreated disease is invariably fatal. If the disorder is discovered early enough, it can be treated with penicillamine, which promotes the excretion of copper, and which must be taken for life. A low dose of penicillamine taken for only two weeks, however, caused neurological deterioration in a 28-year-old man diagnosed with Wilson's disease. Treatment was changed to zinc sulphate, and most of his symptoms improved slowly in the following four years.[328]

In order to prevent further copper accumulation, foods high in copper (organ meats, shellfish, nuts, dried legumes, chocolate, and whole grain cereals) must not be eaten.[329]

* * *

As we have seen, there are several diseases that can impair memory. But they are very rare. Even AD, a scourge that worries most older people, will affect very few of them under a very advanced age. On the other hand, AAMI affects almost all of us, to some degree, as we age. Fortunately, it can be treated.

11

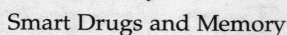

Smart Drugs and Memory

Nootropic drugs

◆

Amino acids

◆

Melatonin

◆

Deprenyl: An MAO inhibitor

◆

Nimodipine

◆

Cognex and Aricept

◆

Be Smart About Drugs

A s we write this, huge amounts of money are being spent by large pharmaceutical companies worldwide on "smart-drug" research. To date, however, except for PS, no nutritional-supplement, prescription, or non-prescription drug has been proven to be both truly effective and without significant side effects in treating AAMI.

MEMORY MOMENT _____

ENHANCED LEARNING WITH DRUGS

he earliest attempts to show that drugs could influence learning were conducted by Dr. K. S. Lashley in 1917 when he demonstrated that low doses of strychnine, a known poison, given to rats before daily training increased their rate of maze learning, although obviously this is not recommended for humans.

Nevertheless, there are some straws in the wind—and quite a few groundless rumors—about prescription drugs that are said to be effective. In this chapter, therefore, we shall discuss which pharmaceuticals may, eventually, lead the way to improved therapies.

Please note, we are not recommending any of these drugs. This would apply even if we were your own physicians, and even if all these drugs were available in this country (many of them are not). We wouldn't recommend them because Dr. Crook has knowledge of most of them through his research organization. And to date, no magic bullet has emerged.

With this broad caveat, let us mention a few of the main "smart drugs" that do exist here or outside the United States and explain why they are thought to have some efficacy.

Nootropic Drugs

PIRACETAM

Nootropics, a word derived from the Greek meaning "towards the mind," are drugs categorized by their chemical composition. One class of nootropics is derived from pyrrolidone, a substance that is said to increase the nervous system's efficiency in using acetylcholine as a neurotransmitter. The drugs in this class include *piracetam* and its analogs (similar molecular structure) oxiracetam, aniracetam, and pramiracetam.[330] It is said that piracetam may enhance the integration of information processing, and improve attention span and concentration.[331] There is also a bit of evidence that suggests it may increase the number of receptors in the brain, especially at the synaptic gap[332] and especially for the cholinergic and dopaminergic pathways. When older mice (18 months) were given large doses of piracetam for two weeks, they developed a 30 to 40 percent higher density of cholinergic receptors in their frontal cortexes than before treatment. The same dosage did not, however, affect four-week-old mice.[333]

According to another theory, piracetam *seems* to improve the blood flow in the brain, increasing the brain's use of sugar (glucose) and oxygen. Some studies suggest that it enhances protein syntheses in the brain, an action essential to the laying down of long-term memory. Others believe its major benefit is that it enhances the function of the nerve fibers in the corpus callosum, thereby increasing the flow of information from the right and left hemispheres of the brain.[334] However, there is no definitive evidence. A Russian study suggested that it reduces free radicals and may have antioxidant properties.[335]

One of the problems with studying smart drugs such as piracetam is that there is a great deal of flawed research published. On quick reading, this research seems to support the drug under review. But more careful perusal of the research often shows that it was self-serving. For example, a study conducted in France showed that the combined use of piracetam plus cognitive-therapy training was more effective than piracetam alone with a group of patients with age-associated memory impairment, and was more effective at a higher dosage of piracetam (4.8 grams as opposed to 2.4 grams). If you read these results carefully, however, you will note that they prove that *cognitive therapy* works, not piracetam.[336]

Of course, piracetam is not the only culprit when it comes to questionable research. Many drugs are researched for marketing, *not* scientific purposes. Throughout this book, we have tried not to be misled by such flawed or biased investigations.

Getting back to piracetam itself, and putting aside the questionable research, we conclude that there may be some benefit, in certain circumstances, such as reading skills in dyslexic children[337]; restoring language after a stroke[338]; and treating people with hypertension who were working under conditions of stress.[339]

However, the results with patients with Alzheimer's disease have been mixed, sometimes showing slight improvements in alertness or certain memory tasks and at other times showing little effect.[340]

At present, piracetam is not sold in the U.S. A 1994 review of the 407 studies published from 1965 to 1992 on piracetam and piracetam-like nootropics (oxiracetam, pramiracetam, etiracetam, nefiracetam, aniracetam, and rolziracetam) reported that piracetam has a very low toxicity level and "lacks serious side effects."[341]

HYDERGINE

Hydergine (generically known as ergoloid mesylates) is made from the ergot fungus of rye plants and was discovered by chemist Albert Hofmann, better known for his discovery of another ergot derivative, LSD 25. It has been available in the United States for more than twenty years, but as a drug that requires a doctor's prescription.

There is limited evidence that Hydergine may act in several ways to enhance mental abilities and to slow down or reverse the aging processes in the brain.[342] The mechanisms behind the drug's ability to do so continue to be studied, but a review of clinical trials reported that Hydergine had been widely tested including in a study of 1,300 patients and on balance, shown to be somewhat effective for improving cerebral metabolism, intellect, and memory.[343] It is believed that Hydergine increases the quantities of blood and oxygen that reach the brain and increases metabolism in brain cells. It may also increase the production of the neurotransmitters dopamine and norepinephrine, which, you may recall from earlier chapters, are essential to the formation of memories. Finally, Hydergine may also help stabilize the brain's metabolism of glucose, thus enhancing both concentration and memory.

However, there are many contradictory studies about this complicated chemical. For example, a 1997 U.S. double-blind study of outpatients aged 55 to 80 years old with mild memory impairment showed that, according to their physicians' rating of memory, the 22 who took Hydergine for 12 weeks showed significant improvement of memory compared to the 19 individuals taking a placebo. On the other hand, structured tests of recent memory showed equal improvement in both groups.[344]

Hydergine has been approved by the FDA for the treatment of senile dementia and insufficient blood circulation to the brain. In Europe it also can be used preventively with patients who have mild mental deterioration. It is an over-the-counter medication in Mexico.

The U.S.-approved dosage is 3 milligrams per day; the

European recommended dosage is 9 milligrams per day taken in three divided doses. Much of the research on Hydergine has been done using 9 to 12 milligrams per day. Side effects include nausea, gastric disturbance, and headache, which may disappear with continued ingestion of the drug, but it may take several weeks before Hydergine produces notable effects on cognition. Hydergine's original patent has expired, so now several generic versions are available.

In our judgment, Hydergine is a mild mood-elevating agent that lets people feel somewhat more sanguine about their memory abilities. Thus, they report AAMI declines. However, when measured objectively, Hydergine seems to result in very little if any actual memory improvement.

Amino Acids

ACETYL-L-CARNITINE

Acetyl-L-carnitine (ALCAR) is a derivative of carnitine, which is found in meat and milk, but not in vegetables. Usually considered an amino acid because its chemical structure is similar, actually it is a substance related to the B vitamins.[345] Acetyl-L-carnitine is distributed throughout the brain and, acting as an antioxidant, appears to counteract certain free radicals and oxidative lesions that accumulate with age. This may reverse some age-associated deficits.[346] Acetyl-L-carnitine has been available in Italy since 1986, but it is not available in the United States.

◆ **Age-Associated Memory Impairment.** A randomized, double-blind study of 15 patients of both sexes, ages 65 +, suffering from mild mental impairment, underwent either therapy with acetyl-L-carnitine (2 grams daily) or took a placebo for three months. Those on the acetyl-L-carnitine improved significantly more in memory, attention, verbal fluency, and daily behavior compared to those taking the placebo.[347] Subsequently, some of the same group of researchers followed a larger randomized group of 30 patients, each with the same results.[348]

◆ **Cerebrovascular Insufficiency.** Reduced blood flow to the brain is a common problem in aging as atherosclerosis causes blood vessels to become too narrow to supply blood to the brain. In a double-blind, crossover study where 12 elderly people undergoing rehabilitation for cerebrovascular insufficiency took acetyl-L-carnitine for part of the study and a placebo for another phase, significant differences were found in favor of the drug on memory, number, and word tests, on maze-drawing performance, and in response to simple stimuli.[349]

◆ **Treatment of Alzheimer's Patients.** Autopsies of the brains of Alzheimer's patients show a significant decrease in the catalyst that produces acetyl-L-carnitine.[350] Therefore, using acetyl-L-carnitine for a lengthy period with probable Alzheimer's disease patients should result in significantly lowered deterioration. This thesis was tested in a study of 20 patients in a 24-week randomized, double-blind, placebo-controlled clinical trial.[351] However, at the end of the test, there was no statistical difference between the test patients and the placebo recipients. Nausea and/or vomiting occurred in five of the seven patients in the acetyl-L-carnitine group.[352]

◆ In a one-year, double-blind, placebo-controlled, randomized multicenter study conducted by researchers at the University of California at San Diego School of Medicine, people aged 50 or older, with mild to moderate probable AD, were treated with three grams a day of

> 66 The charm, one might say the genius of
> memory, is that it is choosy, chancy, and
> temperamental: it rejects the edifying cathedral and
> indelibly photographs the small boy outside, chewing a
> hunk of melon in the dust."
> —Elizabeth Bowen, twentieth-century Anglo-Irish novelist.

ALCAR for one year. Patients 65 years or younger (called the "early-onset" subgroup) declined more slowly with ALCAR than those on a placebo. But the same degree of improvement did not appear to apply to patients over 66.[353]

On balance, then, ALCAR seems to have some limited benefits on AD, but its effect on AAMI are unknown, and the drug may have significant potential side effects.

Melatonin

Melatonin is the principal hormone produced by the pineal gland. Largely thought to be insignificant until recently, the pineal gland is now known to be important in the regulation of hormone balances and circadian rhythms and in maintaining the integrity of the immune system. The disorganization of circadian rhythms is a hallmark of aging and may be related to the progressive deterioration of memory functions. In experimental animals, disruption of circadian rhythms produces retrograde amnesia by interfering with the circadian organization of memory processes. The human circadian system is synchronized to a 24-hour cycle via light that travels by a neural pathway from the retina of the eye to a part of the anterior hypothalamus known as the *supra chiasmatic nucleus.*

Melatonin levels remain low during the day, and at sunset the pineal gland begins releasing melatonin, which peaks at about 2 A.M. As we age, the release of melatonin not only decreases in intensity, but begins later in the evening. Thus, melatonin causes phase shifts in our circadian rhythms, reducing core body temperature and inducing drowsiness.

When melatonin release or intensity is disrupted—as in aging, stress, jet lag, night and rotating shift work, blindness, and rare cases of lesions on the pineal gland—many physiological and mental functions are adversely affected.[354] This is when melatonin supplements may assist cognitive or memory functions, although we are not convinced about melatonin's effect on cognitive performance. If anything, the effect of melatonin may be adverse to memory. Researchers in Norway tested one person on four cognitive tests during time of peak melatonin in the blood and found that the hormone had no direct or immediate effect on information processing, but that the speed of cognitive processing was slowed down.[355]

Researchers in Sheffield, England, investigated the effect of melatonin on police officers working spans of seven successive night shifts. When melatonin was taken at the desired bedtime, sleep problems improved and alertness during working hours increased, especially during the early morning. However, memory scanning speed and perception of mental load were adversely affected.[356]

In general, then, we do not recommend melatonin except for jet lag, agreeing with Ward Dean that "When taken in opposition to the body's natural circadian rhythm, [melatonin can] cause cognitive deficit just like jet-lag does. But when taken in synchronization with the body's natural circadian rhythms, they enhance mental performance."[357]

Deprenyl: An MAO Inhibitor

L-deprenyl, more conveniently just called deprenyl (brand names Selegiline, Elderpryl, Jumex, Movergan), is an MAO-B inhibitor used primarily to treat Parkinson's disease. It alters the neurotransmission of monoamines. Monoamine oxidase enzymes (MAO) are found throughout the body and come in Type A and Type B, the latter being found predominantly in brain glial cells. The activity of this enzyme significantly increases with age.[358] Increased MAO levels are thought to be associated with depression, and for many years drugs that inhibit MAO have been used as antidepressants.

Deprenyl, developed by Professor József Knoll of Semmelweis University in Budapest, Hungary,[359] is readily absorbed from the gastrointestinal tract, and is claimed to correct age-related decreases in certain neurotransmitters, especially dopamine, and therefore to facilitate access to long-term memory inaccessible because of neurotransmitter dysfunction. In controversial studies, it has been shown to extend the maximum lifespan in rats by about 40 percent,[360] and to slow by three months the age-related decline of one form of long-term memory in hamsters.[361]

Deprenyl and Alzheimer's Disease

The results of deprenyl on AD are, at best, mixed. In a controlled trial, doctors at the Bronx Veterans Hospital in New York gave L-deprenyl to 15 outpatients with Alzheimer's disease. In random order, patients received the drug for a four-week period and a placebo for another four weeks. During both periods their cognitive performance was assessed. Although the deprenyl produced no side effects, it also did not significantly improve cognition for digit span, verbal fluency, list learning, delayed recall, and delayed recognition tasks.[362]

Yet in a double-blind, randomized trial conducted in Italy and lasting six months, deprenyl was shown to make a significant difference in information-processing abilities and learning strategies in patients with Alzheimer's disease.[363] The same group of researchers also looked at the effect of deprenyl on the memory of Alzheimer patients in the early stage of their disease. In a six-month, randomized, double-blind, crossover study, they analyzed the drug's influence on the verbal memory of 19 early-onset Alzheimer's patients. The results showed significantly better performances for L-deprenyl–treated patients in learning and long-term memory skills than when the placebo was administered.[364]

A recent study sponsored by the National Institute on Aging suggested that deprenyl, as well as vitamin E, may slightly slow the deterioration of AD.

Because it is used for the treatment of both Parkinson's and Alzheimer's diseases, where it improves attention and episodic memory,[365] deprenyl is available in the U.S. with a doctor's prescription.

❖ MEMORY MOMENT _____

66 *E veryone complains of his memory, and no one complains of his judgment."*
—François, Duc de La Rochefoucauld, seventeenth-century French moralist.

Nimodipine

Nimodipine is a calcium-channel blocker, a kind of drug often used for hypertension, migraine headaches, epilepsy, angina pains, and congestive heart failure. Sold in the U.S. under the brand names Nimotop and Periplum, nimodipine acts to alter the flow of calcium ions through cell membranes. By doing so, it increases blood flow in the brain by preventing constriction of blood vessels, thus lessening oxygen deprivation to brain cells.[366] Nimodipine has also been shown to increase acetylcholine levels in young rats.[367]

In a multicenter, placebo-controlled, double-blind clinical study conducted through Vanderbilt University in Nashville, Tennessee, treatment with 90 milligrams of nimodipine administered in three divided doses for 12 weeks was significantly superior to a placebo on tests of memory, depression, and general state of mind.[368] However, this is isolated evidence and hardly qualifies nimodipine as a smart drug, particularly as other students have shown no comparable effects.

Nimodipine appears to have few if any side effects, is approved in the U.S. for treatment of hemorrhagic stroke, and is being investigated for treatment of patients with Alzheimer's disease.

Cognex and Aricept

These prescription drugs have now been approved by the FDA for treating AD. It is possible that they could also have beneficial effects on AAMI.

However, Cognex has toxic side effects on the liver of some patients. While this is an acceptable risk relative to the greater risk of AD, it is likely that it is not appropriate, even for study, for AAMI.

Aricept has a far better side-effect profile and therefore merits study to determine its effect on AAMI. Since it is on the market, it can presently be prescribed by physicians for AAMI, although we are not aware how broadly this is happening.

Be Smart About Drugs

For those who may be able to find smart drugs outside the U.S. or who have a doctor willing to write a prescription so you can use them for cognitive-enhancing purposes, rather than the purposes for which they were approved or studied, we urge you to use them *only* under the supervision of a physician. And we urge you, too, to get a second opinion. Not infrequently, doctors (being human) who prescribe a given drug believe in it so firmly that they become biased in their evaluation. This happens especially when they see an impressive improvement in one or two patients and ascribe it to the drug in question. Unfortunately, such observations mean nothing in the absence of scientifically established controls. They could easily have occurred by pure coincidence.

Also, while some of the drugs discussed in this chapter appear to be free from adverse side effects, the combination of them with other drugs, and possibly with nutritional supplements, is unknown and could be harmful.

Since the publication of many of the books on brain-boosting drugs, and the "underground" popularity of the drugs, the FDA, which once allowed small supplies of nonapproved drugs to be imported or mailed into this country for personal use, has begun a crackdown of the best-known sources, making it extremely difficult to get them in the United States for other than prescribed purposes.

Although this chapter has explored some of the research available on "smart drugs" that have been developed and are available for various uses, it is by no means meant as a user's guide to advocate the use of these drugs. Indeed, we believe *The Memory Cure* shows you that, by using phosphatidylserine, you will be taking a legal, safe, probably less expensive, and certainly more effective way to improve your memory.

12

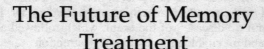

The Future of Memory Treatment

Now where did I leave that memory?

◆

New tests make for more effective diagnoses

◆

Growing technology expands our knowledge

◆

Brain cell regeneration: An exciting lead

◆

What does sex have to do with it?

◆

The future of PS

◆

Looking forward

❖

We've come a long way since the seventeenth-century German psychiatrist Emil Kraepelin coined the term "paramnesia" for what he called "errors of memory." Dr. Kraepelin had no thought that anything physical might be involved. Rather, he thought the "errors" were thought deceptions, although not necessarily done with malicious intent. We had to wait until the nineteenth century for the French psychologist Théodule-Armand Ribot to entertain the notion that memory loss could be the result of something physiological. Dr. Ribot called it a "disease" of the brain, which followed a specific and inevitable progression of destruction.

Now Where Did I Leave That Memory?

From the early days of the neurosciences, the notion that memory is located in a specific structure of the brain has been prevalent. In the eighteenth century, a school of psychology called "phrenology" emerged, which held that the brain could be separated into different centers, each controlling a separate behavior process. Phrenologists drew maps of the skull showing the exact locations of the 37 "powers of the mind." Although there was no physical basis for phrenology, nineteenth-century physicians also proposed the existence of many centers in the brain that controlled specific behaviors.

Then along came an American neurophysiologist by the name of Karl Lashley, who studied brain functions in laboratory animals for more than 30 years. Dr. Lashley came to the then-radical conclusion that memory didn't appear to be located in any single region of the cortex.[369] Following in Lashley's footsteps, scientists have continued to make great strides in uncovering the intricately complicated nature of the memory process, especially with respect to aging. In 1960 there were only 3,222 Americans over the age of 100.[370] Today that number has increased to 60,000. As the number of aging persons in our population continues to spiral upward, researchers, likewise, have turned their attention to the relationship between aging and memory, and doubtless that area of study will continue to expand.

We're certain that by now you have an understanding that memory is much more complicated—and a much more active process—than any of the pioneers into memory research understood or even imagined. There are a number of factors other than AAMI that affect memory, several of which may result in problems that are so similar that they are often misdiagnosed. As more and more people get the message that AAMI does not mean that they are likely to sink rapidly into AD, they may be able to reduce their anxiety and improve their memory accordingly. We have seen how the results of stress can mimic some cognitive disorders and unnecessarily frighten millions of older people.

Research centers all over the world are developing programs to study memory and cognition, and are seeking ways to treat AD, AAMI, and other cognitive disorders. For instance, researchers at Park Research Lab in Ann Arbor, Michigan, are investigating the mechanisms that account for age-related differences in memory decline[371] and are attempting to determine how deeply cultural differences may influence basic cognitive and human information-processing strategies and biases.[372] Some members of the research team are examining age-related differences in controlling attention,[373] while others are working to clarify the combined effects of alcohol and aging on cognition.[374] A new line of research in the Park Lab will focus on how older adults' perceptions of aging affects their own cognitive performance.[375]

New Tests Make for More Effective Diagnoses

Researchers at institutions nationwide are refining the definitions of exactly what constitutes AD, AAMI, or

❖ MEMORY MOMENT _____

> 66 I lliterate him, I say, quite from your
> memory."
>
> —Mrs. Malaprop in Richard Brinsley
> Sheridan's *The Rivals*.

other age-associated memory disorders. As a result, we shall be able to understand the problem of AAMI better in the future. Until the last few years, most treatment research has been devoted to finding cures for AD. Less effort has been devoted to nondisease-related memory decline. That is where we must turn next, for many of us no longer accept AAMI as inevitable.

Growing Technology Expands Our Knowledge

The use of new methodologies and techologies now allow us to understand and even visualize changes in brain function that occur with advanced age. A new brain imaging machine called an fMRI (functional Magnetic Resonance Imaging) allows researchers to pinpoint ever more clearly which areas of the brain are involved in different types of memory, as well as speech, and other cognitive processes. This new equipment has sharper resolution than machines used in the past and doesn't require that any radioactive tracers be injected into a person in order to view brain activity. Not only can the use of brain mapping by the fMRI tell us more about how the brain works, but it will also enable us to determine whether there is another part of the brain that can take over for areas that have been damaged by stroke, accident, tumors, or other disorders.[376]

Nearly half of the ongoing research at the Salk Institute for Biological Studies is concentrated on the brain. In the Salk's Cognitive Neuroscience Laboratory, investigators under the leadership of Dr. Ursula Belligi are using high-speed computers to produce three-dimensional images of living brains from two-dimensional magnetic resonance imaging (MRI) data. In this way they can directly visualize, examine, and compare the various regions of the brain that are active in language, spatial abilities, memory, and other cognitive functions to determine how they are affected in people with neurological disorders or injuries.[377]

Brain Cell Regeneration: An Exciting Lead

In the Salk's Molecular Neurobiology Laboratory, Professor Stephen Heinemann is investigating a gene therapy approach to introducing molecules known at present only as "free radical scavengers." Their function would be to "soak up" and neutralize free radicals, those toxic entities that result in cell death.[378]

Within the last decade, scientists discovered that the growth of new dendritic branches can be stimulated by "nerve growth factor" (NGF), a group of powerful brain chemicals, only some of which have yet been identified. Researchers in Sweden have transplanted nerve cells, genetically engineered to secrete nerve growth factor into various sections of the brains of aged rats and have subsequently found increased NGF tissue content for at least 10 weeks after grafting.[379] If a similar approach proves broadly feasible in humans (a big question, of course), it may provide an entirely new path to brain—and memory—repair and regeneration.

One area of considerable controversy—and one that you will hear much more about in coming years thanks to a landmark study conducted at Princeton University in New Jersey and published in 1998—is the question of whether or not our brain cells can regenerate, a process previously thought impossible. The idea that they might was first supported by research showing that new neurons continue to grow in adult fish and birds. One of the early studies of this kind was reported in a 1984 article in *Science*.[380] When Fernando Nottebohm and his colleagues at Rockefeller University studied canaries, they found up to a 40 percent loss of neurons after the breeding season, but new neuronal growth after the fall when the birds learn new songs for the next breeding season. It appears that the new cycle of learning songs stimulated the birds' brains to form new neurons in a specialized area in the canary brain that responds to sound.[381]

These experiments were thought to have little implication for humans and were largely ignored until neurologist Elizabeth Gould at Princeton examined six marmoset monkeys whose brains had been injected with a chemical to mark cells that divided or regenerated. Later, the monkeys were injected with a different chemical to mark mature brain cells; hence, new cells that had matured would carry the marks of both chemicals. Dr. Gould's research team reported significant new cellular growth in the hippocampus of the monkeys' brains.[382] Such increased cell quantity should, in theory, greatly enhance memory.

What Does Sex Have to Do with It?

The new imaging technologies have awakened us to the fact that men lose brain cells three times as fast as women do. Although the brains of males are larger in youth, by middle age they have come to be about the same size as that of females. Men generally have thicker, more developed right hemispheres and typically perform better than women on visual-spatial tasks of memory. Women, who have more developed left hemispheres, outperform men on tests of verbal fluency and do better on remembering details.[383] In navigating through the world, men have more of a sense of a spatial map in their mind ("Go so far this way and then turn left"). Women pay attention to and use landmarks to guide them.

These differences may be, in part, due to hormones. Several controlled clinical studies of the administration of estrogen to postmenopausal women have found that estrogen enhances verbal memory and helps maintain the ability to learn new material. The author of one of the studies, Dr. B. B. Sherwin, speculates that it may well be that in adulthood, estrogen activates neural pathways in women that were already established under its influence during prenatal life.[384] Estrogen also increases the production of the neurotransmitters acetylcholine and stimulates a significant increase in dopamine receptors in the brain.[385]

An "iffy" and as yet unresolved question with regard to memory in aging women is whether or not estrogen-replacement therapy (ERT) has a protective effect on cognitive function in postmenopausal women. A number of studies seem to suggest that it does, and that it may do this by stimulating the action of certain neurotransmitters.[386] However, other studies have produced contrary results, so the matter remains in dispute.

Estrogen boosts the production of acetylcholine and impedes the deposit of beta-amyloid, the protein believed to be involved in the characteristic plaques of Alzheimer's disease. In one of the most remarkable findings to date, a 16-year study by scientists at the National Institute on Aging at Johns Hopkins Bayview Medical Center showed that a history of ERT in women after menopause was associated with close to a 50 percent reduction in the risk of developing Alzheimer's disease.[387]

Estrogen may also improve blood flow and helps maintain the integrity of the hippocampus. When some of the same researchers in the preceding study compared 116 postmenopausal women who were receiving ERT with 172 women who had never received ERT, those who were taking the hormone showed fewer errors on a measure of short-term visual memory and on visual perception. Furthermore, ERT appeared to protect against age changes in a subgroup of 18 women for whom memory scores were available before and during ERT treatment.[388]

Prior to the 1997 report of the 16-year study cited above, researchers at Yale University School of Medicine reviewed 19 studies related to estrogen and cognition. All the studies were published between 1970 and 1996 in English-language publications. Of the 10 randomized trials of ERT versus placebo, eight claimed therapeutic benefits, and three reported significant improvements in memory and/or attention. The other nine studies were considered "observational" (meaning strict research protocols were not used). Five found a significant association between estrogen use and cognitive function. The reviewers concluded that, while the observational studies provided encouraging leads, there was still not enough evidence from randomized, controlled studies to provide a definitive answer.[389] Thus, large placebo-controlled trials are still required to address estrogen's role in the prevention and treatment of AAMI and AD.

Until then, given that estrogen does carry certain risks with it, we do not feel we can recommend estrogen for the treatment of AAMI or AD.[390] However, we hope new research will be forthcoming soon because we believe this is likely to be a fruitful path for investigation.

The Future of PS

Listen to what Parris Kidd, Ph.D., probably the most knowledgeable researcher about PS in the world, has to say about PS:

> The list of potential applications for PS is constantly being expanded. First, it satisfies an essential prerequisite for a healing substance: do no harm. Being intrinsic to the body's biochemistry, PS is extremely safe for everyone to take, no matter how old or how sick. Second, PS is extremely versatile in its clinical effects. Found in all cells from the most primitive all the way through to those of humans, PS acts at such a profound level of the living cell that it benefits virtually any brain function that is less than optimal. Third, PS is well validated through clinical research.
>
> The use of PS is so well tolerated, its track record so unblemished, its potency as a brain nutrient so real, that it will remain on the cutting edge of brain research. Without doubt, further clinical study will open up ever more exciting avenues of application for PS.

Dr. Kidd has also stated that PS is close to being an ideal agent for use in combination with other orally administered healing substances. To start with, PS preparations have the natural emulsifying action typical of lecithin-phospholipid mixtures. This action aids in dispersing foodstuffs in the intestine, and is likely to improve the absorption of nutrients that are administered together with PS. These qualities make PS a natural choice for use in combination with other nutrients. In the future PS will be routinely employed in combination with vitamins, minerals, semi-essential nutrients, and certain herbal preparations, all of which ought to help further optimize the remarkable benefits of PS.

Looking Forward

Although the loss of mental and physical capacities in the later decades of life was once thought to be inevitable, we now know that there are a variety of things each of us can do to help prevent this in our own lives. And further research promises even more help in this respect in the coming years.

Dr. David Snowdon's ongoing study of the Minnesota nuns (see Chapter 10), most of whom live full, productive, and happy lives well into their nineties, will surely tell us more about the "successful aging" process. The nuns have agreed to donate their brains to Dr. Snowdon at the University of Kentucky's Sanders-Brown Center on Aging. Although some of them have Alzheimer's, Dr. Snowdon has already discovered that this particular group of nuns has less Alzheimer's than the general population. He continues to seek answers as to how this might apply to the rest of us.

A number of training programs have shown that adopting mnemonic techniques, such as our Memory Maximizer exercises in Chapter 5, can also improve everyday memory tasks. Maintaining your health in the various ways described throughout this book can not only prevent memory decline, but mitigate already existing problems. Ongoing developments in neurochemistry and pharmacology have developed compounds that, probably in conjunction with PS, will eventually be used to control or reverse the age-related changes underlying AAMI.

The "first generation" of these drugs continues to be evaluated, and others will undoubtedly follow.

Now let us join Dr. Kidd again as he looks into the slightly more distant future and sees a fundamental change in how we shall treat mental and memory impairment:

PS for Rejuvenating Declining Brain Power

The first decade of the 21st century will see the emergence of "Brain Power" clinics around the United States and elsewhere on the planet. Such clinics will have a thriving business in evaluating, diagnosing, and counseling citizens with a view to correcting their brain flaws in order to help them optimize their performance on the job and in social settings. The clinics will be organized something like this:

As you enter the clinic, you will be asked to fill out a questionnaire that will include questions on whether you smoke, drink alcohol regularly, have used cocaine or other illegal drugs (including marijuana). The questionnaire will also probe your consumption of sleep aids, anti-depressants, or other legal mind-altering drugs, many of which cause memory loss and other symptoms that resemble dementia. Some of these people will be routed to a High-Risk Memory Loss Clinic.

Those of us who have taken good enough care of ourselves to clear this first hurdle will next have our cognitive performance assessed (especially learning, concentration, memory, word recall) using computer and video neuropsychological tests similar to the ones Dr. Crook currently administers. Following the assessment, the technicians will consult tables and charts, then tell you how "normal" or close to "optimal" your performance measured, as compared with the rest of the population on age-, gender-, and culture-matched bias. There will be cut-off points for performance, below which you will be judged "atypical" or "hypofunctional" or "at risk for dementia." Dr. Crook has been a pioneer in this area and his tests have continuously advanced the state-of-the-art in neuropsychological testing for the past two decades.

If you didn't score so well and are assigned to one of these categories, you may have to be further evaluated through real-time brain scanning (Positron Emission Tomography—PET—or something like it). You'll be able to see your brain light up on a screen in real time, as it burns a labeled "energy substrate" for the energy it needs to function. Depending on how well your brain is found to burn the labeled glucose or phosphate sample that they feed to you, and depending on which brain zones are most hypofunctional, you will either be referred to a dementia specialist for further diagnostic workup, or the technicians will pass you on to a Brain Nutrition Specialist in the same clinic. This licensed professional will assess your dietary habits, suggest ways to optimize your diet, then give you a list of nutrients you should be taking to supplement your diet.

Finally, prior to leaving the clinic you will be seen by a physician who will summarize for you the findings from the Brain Risk questionnaire, the Brain Performance Evaluation, the Brain Metabolic Scan, the Brain Nutrient Status assessment, and whatever other information you choose to disclose. The physician will advise you of your options for optimizing areas of brain function that seemed hypofunctional. He or she will explain why you are being prescribed PS and why it may be necessary to add in other nutrients or even drugs to this regimen. You will also be advised how to best meditate and practice breathing exercises, and why you should clean up your home and work environment to minimize further exposure to toxic influences.

There you have it, the future unveiled! If you want to learn more, Brenda Adderly's newsletter, *Health Watch*, will keep you up to date with this rapidly unfolding field. For more information on memory, or to test your memory abilities, visit Dr. Crook's website (www.psychologix.com). *But* most important of all . . .

<u>You Don't Have to Wait</u>

As positive as the thought of these new developments is, you don't have to wait for FDA approval of prescription drugs or decades-long research studies to enhance a failing memory. PS may be the first of an entire generation of substances to limit or reverse the effects of aging. The life-improving benefits of phosphatidylserine are available to you now. No longer do you have to worry that you are on the road to steady mental decline. You now know the steps you can take. By following *The Memory Cure,* you have a simple and effective means of rejuvenating your memory functions. You don't have to wait another day to reap the benefits of improving your brain's ability to effectively send along its messages . . . and thus to improve your life.

AFTERWORD TO THE PAPERBACK PUBLICATION

Since the publication of *The Memory Cure* in mid-1998, thousands of people have successfully turned back the clock on memory loss by taking the nutritional supplement phosphatidylserine (PS) and following our recommended program. And as exciting and effective as PS is for halting age-related memory loss, additional revolutionary breakthroughs with PS are now coming to light.

Having recognized PS's ability to improve general brain functioning, the scientific community is now looking into the supplement's effects beyond memory, and into cognitive function as a whole as it relates to stress. To that end, the ability of PS to enhance overall mental and physical performance is being explored by researchers around the world.

Thomas Crook, Ph.D., the coauthor of this book, is spearheading the research initiative into mental performance for people of all ages. Specifically, a study is currently under way with a selected and screened group of college students at a major university to test the hypothesis that PS can help improve a person's performance under highly stressful conditions, like a difficult exam. If the results prove positive, the broad ramifications for anyone working in a stressful environment are extraordinary. Imagine the value to society of a dietary supplement that can enhance the performance of our police officers, firemen, and surgeons, just to name a few. And imagine what a huge benefit it would be to every student if PS could reduce their pre-exam stress and allow them to study more productively before their exam, and therefore perform better.

PS and Athletic Performance

Concurrently, a number of studies have now been completed to determine whether PS can enhance physical performance. During intense physical exertion, the body reacts to "stress" by increasing the amount of cortisol, a stress hormone, which tends to inhibit performance. Testosterone, on the other hand, is another hormone produced during exercise that has a positive effect on body chemistry and actually increases muscle, which in turn has a salutary effect on athletic performance. An athlete, therefore, wishes to minimize the muscle-depleting effects of cortisol while maximizing the effects of testosterone.

Three recent studies have shown that PS supplementation may inhibit exercise-induced increases in cortisol without the side effects of anabolic steroids, carbohydrate drinks, protein bars and other muscle-enhancing products.[391]

In one of these studies[392], conducted at the University of Naples in Italy, researchers found that taking PS can lessen the severity of the stress response to exercise, and thus improve athletic performance. Healthy, nonathletic males took either 50 or 75 mg of PS and then bicycled to near exhaustion. Blood samples were taken before, during, and after the exercise. As expected, cortisol levels rose after this intense exercise, but compared to the placebo trial, the increase was 33 percent *less* when the subjects took 50 mg of PS and 45 percent less when they took 75 mg.

These same Italian researchers conducted a followup experiment with an oral daily dose of 400 or 800 mg of PS (or a placebo) for ten days prior to exercise. The research team found that the cortisol response to exercise was about 16 percent lower for the 400 mg dose and 30 percent lower for the 800 mg dose, when compared to the placebo. This further convinced researchers that, in healthy people, PS can significantly reduce the impact of the stress response to exercise.[393]

In a U.S. study[394] at California State University, Chico, researchers found cortisol levels to be 20 percent lower in subjects who ingested PS. In their double-blind crossover study, researchers measured the effects of 800 mg of PS taken daily during a two-week intense weight-training regimen as compared to a placebo. The subjects did five sets of 10 repetitions of 13 exercises four times per week. The researchers wanted to exhaust the subjects and overtrain their muscles, similar to the regimen professional athletes endure. They found that cortisol levels were indeed lower in those who took the PS supplement. Also, exit interviews showed that the subjects taking PS had a significantly better perception of well-being, had less muscle soreness, and their perceived level of exertion dropped.

While these results are still preliminary, they do offer another exciting aspect to ongoing phosphatidylserine research. Once more definitive studies have taken place, PS may prove to be an essential phospholipid for people of all ages who wish to improve brain or physical functions.

We hope you enjoy using the preceeding information on your brain, memory, PS, and how to keep yourself mentally sharp for a lifetime as you embark on The Memory Cure.

—December 1998

NOTES

1. Youngjohn, J. R., G. J. Larrabee, and T. H. Crook. First-Last Names and the Grocery List Selective Reminding Test: Two Computerized Measures of Everyday Verbal Learning. *Archives of Clinical Neuropsychology* 6: 287–300 (1991).
2. Crook, T. H., G. Zappala, et al. Republic of San Marino Normal Population Sampling, *Developmental Neuropsychology* 9(2): 103–113 (1993).
3. Schacter, D. L. *Searching for Memory: The Brain, the Mind, and the Past.* New York: Basic Books, 1996.
4. Graham, K. S., J. T. Becker, and J. R. Hodges. On the Relationship Between Knowledge and Memory for Pictures: Evidence from the Study of Patients with Semantic Dementia and Alzheimer's Disease. *Journal of the International Neuropsychological Society* 3(6): 534–544 (1997).
5. Parkin, A. J. Human Memory: Novelty, Association, and the Brain. *Current Biology* 7(12): R768–R769 (1997).
6. Haxby, J. V., L. G. Ungerleider, B. Horwitz, J. M. Maisog, S. I. Rapoport, and C. L. Grady. Face Encoding and Recognition in the Human Brain. *Proceedings of the National Academy of Sciences of the United States of America* 93(2): 922–927 (Jan. 23, 1996).
7. Zola-Morgan, S. M. and L. R. Squire. The Primate Hippocampal Formation: Evidence for a Time-limited Role in Memory Storage. *Science* 250 (4978): 288–290 (Oct. 12, 1990).

8. Jarrard, L. E. On the Role of the Hippocampus in Learning and Memory in the Rat. *Behavioral and Neural Biology* 60(1): 9–26 (1993).

9. Stuss, D. T., F. I. Craik, L. Sayer, D. Franchi, and M. P. Alexander. Comparison of Older People and Patients with Frontal Lesions: Evidence from Word List Learning. *Psychology and Aging* 11(3): 387–395 (1996).

10. Quillfeldt, J. A., M. S. Zanatta, P. K. Schmitz, J. Quevedo, E. Schaeffer, J. B. Lima, J. H. Medine, and I. Izquierdo. Different Brain Areas are Involved in Memory Expression at Different Times from Training. *Neurobiology of Learning and Memory* 66(2): 97–101 (1996).

11. Brockway, J. P., R. L. Follmer, L. A. Preuss, C. E. Prioleau, G. S. Burrows, K. A. Solsrud, C. N. Cooke, J. H. Greenhoot, and J. Howard. Memory, Simple and Complex Language, and the Temporal Lobe. *Brain and Language* 61(1): 1–29 (1998).

12. Yasuda, K., O. Watanabe, and Y. Ono. Dissociation Between Semantic and Autobiographic Memory: A Case Report. *Cortex* 33(4): 623–638 (1997).

13. Miller, G. A. The Magical Number Seven: Plus or Minus Two. Some Limits on Our Capacity for Processing Information. *The Psychological Review* 9: 81–97 (1956).

14. Gobet, F. and H. A. Simon. Templates in Chess Memory: A Mechanism for Recalling Several Boards. *Cognitive Psychology* 31(1): 1–40 (1996).

15. Schacter, D. L. *Op. cit.*

16. *Ibid.*

17. Higbee, K. L. *Your Memory: How It Works and How to Improve It.* 2d ed. New York: Paragon House, 1988.

18. Terr, L. C. *Unchained Memories.* New York: Basic Books, 1994.

19. Paris, J. Memories of Abuse in Borderline Patients: True or False? *Harvard Review of Psychiatry* 3(1): 10–17 (1995).

20. Edelman, G. *Brilliant Air, Brilliant Fire: On the Matter of the Mind.* New York: Basic Books, 1992.

21. Barclay, C. R. Schematization of Autobiographical Memory. In D. C. Rubin, ed. *Autobiographical Memory.* Cambridge: Cambridge University Press, 1986. 82–99.

22. Samson, J. C. The Biological Basis of Phosphatidylserine Pharmacology. *Clinical Trials Journal* 24(1): 1–8 (1987).

23. *Ibid.*

24. *Advances in Brain Research.* La Jolla: The Salk Institute for Biological Studies, 1996.

25. *Advances in Research on Stroke.* La Jolla: The Salk Institute for Biological Studies, no date.

26. Schacter, D. L. *Op. cit.*

27. Higbee, K. L. *Op. cit.*

28. Squire, L. R. *Memory and Brain.* New York: Oxford University Press, 1987.

29. Schacter, D. L. *Op. cit.*

30. Blakemore, C. and R. C. Van Sluyters. Reversal of the Physiological Effects of Monocular Deprivation in Kittens: Further Evidence for a Sensitive Period. *Journal of Physiology (London)* 237: 195–216 (1974).

31. Olfactory Facts: A Baker's Dozen. *University of California at Berkeley Wellness Letter* 14(7): 3 (April, 1998).

32. Dr. Alan Hirsh. Interviewed by Ivanhoe Broadcast News. Reported on their website *http://www.ivanhoe.com/docs/backissues/braincentsqa.html.*

33. Shadmehr, R. and H. H. Holcomb. Neural Correlates of Motor Memory Consolidation. *Science* 277(5327): 821–825 (8 August 1997).

34. Loftus, E. *Memory: Surprising New Insights into How We Remember and Why We Forget.* Reading, Mass.: Addison-Wesley, 1980.

35. Christianson, S.-Å, and E. F. Loftus. Memory for Traumatic Events. *Applied Cognitive Psychology* 1: 225–223 (1987).

36. Davies, G., and M. Alonso-Quecuty. Cultural Factors in the Recall of a Witnessed Event. *Memory* 5(5): 601–614 (1997).

37. Calev, A. Affect and Memory in Depression: Evidence of Better Delayed Recall of Positive than Negative Affect Words. *Psychopathology* 29(2): 71–76 (1996).

38. Bolla, K. I., K. N. Lindgren, C. Bonaccorsy, and M. L. Bleecker. Memory Complaints in Older Adults. Fact or Fiction? *Archives of Neurology* 48(1): 61–64 (1991).

39. Kimberg, D. Y., M. D'Esposito, and M. J. Farah. Effects of Bromocriptine on Human Subjects Depend on Working Memory Capacity. *Neuroreport* 8(16): 3581, 3585 (1987).

40. Ritchie, K., J. Touchon, B. Ledesert, D. Liebovici, and A. M. Gorce. Establishing the Limits and Characteristics of Normal Age-Related Cognitive Decline. *Revue d' Epidemiologie et de Sante Publique* 45(5), 373–381 (1997). See also Perlmutter, M., R. Metzger, T. Nezworski, and K. Miller. Spatial and Temporal Memory in 20 to 60 Year Olds. *Journal of Gerontology* 36(1), 59–65 (1981).

41. Small, G. W., A. La Rue, S. Komo, A. Kaplan, and M. A. Mandelkern. Predictors of Cognitive Change in Middle-aged and Older Adults with Memory Loss. *American Journal of Psychiatry* 152(12): 1757–1764 (1995).

42. West, R. L., T. H. Crook, and K. L. Barron. Everyday Memory Performance Across the Life Span: Effects of Age and Noncognitive Individual Differences. *Psychology and Aging* 7(1): 72–82 (1992).

43. Petersen, R. C., G. Smith, E. Kokmen, R. J. Ivnik, and E. G. Tangalow. Memory Function in Normal Aging. *Neurology* 42(2): 396–401 (1992).

44. Christensen, H., A. Korten, A. F. Jorm, A. S. Henderson, R. Scott, and A. J. Mackinnon. Activity Levels and Cognitive Functioning in an Elderly Community Sample. *Age and Aging* 25: 72–80 (1996).

45. Baddeley, A. *Your Memory. A User's Guide.* New York: Macmillan Publishing Co., Inc., 1982.

46. Hoffer, A. and M. Walker. *Smart Nutrients.* Garden City Park, N.Y.: Avery Publishing Group, 1994.

47. Kidd, P. M. *Phosphatidylserine (PS): Number-One Brain Booster.* New Canaan, Conn.: Keats Publishing, 1998.

48. Nizzo, M. C., S. Tegos, A. Gallamini, G. Toffano, A. Polleri, and M. Massarotti. Brain Cortex Phospholipids Liposomes Effects of CSF HVAS, 5-HIAA and on Prolactin and Somatotropin Secretion in Man. *Journal of Neural Transmission* 43: 93–102 (1978).

49. Argentiero, V. and B. Tavolato. Dopamine (DA) and Serotonin Metabolic Levels in the Cerebrospinal Fluid (CSF) in Alzheimer's Presenile Dementia Under Basic Conditions and After Stimulation with Cerebral Cortex Phospholipids (BC-PL). *Journal of Neurology* 224: 53–58 (1980).

50. Toffano, G., A. Battistella, and P. Orlando. Pharmacokinetics of Radiolabelled Brain Phosphatidylserine. *Clinical Trials Journal* 24(1): 18–24 (1987).

51. Kidd, P. M. *Phosphatidylserine: The Nutrient Building Block That Accelerates All Brain Functions and Counters Alzheimer's.* New Canaan, Conn.: Keats Publishing, 1998.

52. Calderini, G., A. C. Bonetti, A. Battistella, F. T. Crews, and G. Toffano. Biochemical Changes of Rat Brain Membranes with Aging. *Neurochemical Research* 8(4): 483–492 (1983).

53. Gower, T. Is There a Magic Memory Bullet? *Esquire,* December 1997, 142.

54. Folch, J. The Chemical Structure of Phosphatidylserine. *Journal of Biological Chemistry* 174: 439–50 (1948).

55. Calderini, G., F. Bellini, A. C. Bonetti, E. Galbiati, D. Guidolin, F. Milan, M. G. Nunzi, R. Rubini, A. Zanotti, and G. Toffano. Pharmacological Properties of Phosphatidylserine in the Ageing Brain. *Clinical Trials Journal* 24(1): 9–17 (1987).

56. Kent, A. Can a Tablet Keep Your Mind Sharp in Middle Age? *Daily Mail,* 4 November 1997, Good Health Section, 41.

57. G. Toffano. The Therapeutic Value of Phosphatidylserine Effect in the Aging Brain. In I. Hanin and G. B. Ansell, eds. *Lecithin: Technological, Biological, and Therapeutic Aspects.* New York: Plenum Press, 1987.

58. Caffarra, P. and V. Santamaria. The Effects of Phosphatidylserine in Patients with Mild Cognitive Decline. *Clinical Trials Journal* 24(1): 109–114 (1987).

59. Granata, Q. and J. DiMichele. Phosphatidylserine in Elderly Patients. An Open Trial. *Clinical Trials Journal* 24(1): 99–103 (1987).

60. Sinforiani, E., C. Agostinis, P. Merlo, S. Gualtieri, M. Mauri, and A. Mancuso. Cognitive Decline in Ageing Brain. Therapeutic Approach with Phosphatidylserine. *Clinical Trials Journal* 24(1): 115–124 (1987).

61. Puca, F. M., M. A. Savarese, and M. G. Minervini. Exploratory Trial of Phosphatidylserine Efficacy in Mildly Demented Patients. *Clinical Trials Journal* 24(1): 94–98 (1987).

62. McNeil, C. *Alzheimer's Disease: Unraveling the Mystery.* National Institutes on Aging. Washington, D.C.: National Institutes of Health Public Information Office.

63. Villardita, C., S. Grioli, G. Salmeri, F. Nicoletti, and G. Pennisi. Multicentre Clinical Trial of Brain Phosphatidylserine in Elderly Patients with Intellectual Deterioration. *Clinical Trials Journal* 24(1): 84–93 (1987).

64. Palmieri, G., R. Palmieri, M. R. Inzoli, G. Lombardi, C. Sottini, B. Tavolato, and B. Giometto. Double-blind Controlled Trial of Phosphatidylserine in Patients with Senile Mental Deterioration. *Clinical Trials Journal* 24(1): 73–83 (1987).

65. Nerozzi, D. Fosfatidilserina e disturbi della memoria nell-anziano. *La Clinica Terapeutica* 120: 399–404 (1987).

66. Amaducci, L. and the Smid Group. Phosphatidylserine in

the Treatment of Alzheimer's Disease: Results of Multi-center Study. *Psychopharmacology Bulletin* 24(1): 130–134 (1988).

67. Crook, T. H., J. Tinklenberg, J. Yesavage, W. Petrie, M. G. Nunzi, and D. C. Massari. Effects of Phosphatidylserine in Age-associated Memory Impairment. *Neurology* 41(5): 644–649 (1991).

68. Crook, T., W. Petrie, C. Wells, and D. C. Massari. Effects of Phosphatidylserine in Alzheimer's Disease. *Psychopharmacology Bulletin* 28(1): 61–66 (1992).

69. Cenacchi, T., T. Bertoldin, C. Farina, M. G. Fiori, G. Crepaldi, and Participating Investigators. Cognitive Decline in the Elderly: A Double-blind, Placebo-controlled Multicenter Study on Efficacy of Phosphatidylserine Administration. *Aging: Clinical and Experimental Research* 5: 123–133 (1993).

70. Gindin, J., M. Novikov, D. Kedar, A. Walter-Ginzberg, S. Nacr, O. Karta, E. Zur, and S. Levi. The Effect of Plant Phosphatidylserine on Age-associated Memory Impairment and Mood in the Functioning Elderly. Unpublished study conducted by researchers at the Geriatric Institute for Education and Research and the Department of Geriatrics at Kaplan Hospital, Rehovot, Israel.

71. Kidd, P. M. *Op. cit.*

72. *Ibid.*

73. Heywood, R., D. D. Cozens, and M. Richold. Toxicology of a Phosphatidylserine Preparation from Bovine Brain (BC-PS). *Clinical Trials Journal* 24(1): 25–32 (1987).

74. Potter, B. A. and S. Orfali. *Brain Boosters*. Berkeley, CA: Ronin Publishing Co., 1993.

75. The Brain Benefits from an Enriched Environment. *Salk Institute Signals* 2(2): 4 (Summer 1997).

76. Wild, R., ed. *The Complete Book of Natural and Medicinal Cures*. Emmaus, Pa.: Rodale Press, 1994.

77. Harman, D. Free Radicals in Aging. *Molecular Cell Biochemistry* 84: 155–161 (1988).

78. Our Vitamin Prescription: The Big Four. *University of California at Berkeley Wellness Letter* 10(4): 1–2 (January 1994).

79. Hoffer, A. and M. Walker. *Op. cit.*

80. Higbee, K. L. *Op. cit.*

81. Craik, F. I. M., M. Byrd, and J. M. Swanson. Patterns of Memory Loss in Three Elderly Samples. *Psychology and Aging* 21(1): 79–86 (1987).

82. Milligan, W. L., D. A. Powell, C. Harley, and E. Furchgott. A Comparison of Physical Health and Psychosocial Variables as Predictors of Reaction Time and Serial Learning Performance in Elderly Men. *Journal of Gerontology* 39(6): 704–710 (1984).

83. Dr. Kenneth R. Pelletier. Interviewed in *Bottom Line Tomorrow* 6(3): 11–13 (March 1998).

84. Pelletier, K. R. *Sound Mind, Sound Body.* New York: Simon & Schuster, 1994.

85. Erber, J. T., L. T. Szuchman, and S. T. Rothberg. Dimensions of Self-report About Everyday Memory in Young and Older Adults. *International Journal of Aging and Human Development* 34(4): 311–323 (1992).

86. Smith, G. E., R. C. Petersen, R. J. Ivnik, J. F. Malec, and E. G. Tangalow. Subjective Memory Complaints, Psychological Distress, and Longitudinal Change in Objective Memory Performance. *Psychology and Aging* 11(2): 272–279 (1996).

87. Hunter, I. M. L. *Memory.* Baltimore: Penguin Books, 1964.

88. West, R. L. and A. Tomer. Everyday Memory Problems of Healthy Older Adults: Characteristics of a Successful Intervention. In Gilmore, G. C., P. J. Whitehouse, and M. L. Wykle, eds. *Memory, Aging, and Dementia.* New York: Springer Publishing Co., 1989. 74–98.

89. Kagan, J. with R. Mount. *The Second Year: The Emergence*

of Self Awareness. Cambridge, Mass.: Harvard University Press, 1981.

90. Burack, O. R. and M. E. Lachman. The Effects of List-making on Recall in Young and Elderly Adults. *Journals of Gerontology.* Series B, *Psychological Sciences and Social Sciences* 51(4): P226–P233 (1996).

91. Fogler, J. Common Memory Traps and How to Avoid Them. *Bottom Line Health* 12(1): 19 (January 1988).

92. Wingfield, A. and E. A. L. Stine. Modeling Memory Processes: Research and Theory on Memory and Aging. In Gilmore, G. C., P. J. Whitehouse, and M. L. Wykle, eds. *Op. cit.*

93. Ormond, J. *Human Learning.* 2d ed. Englewood Cliffs, N.J.: Prentice Hall, 1995.

94. Higbee, K. L. *Op. cit.*

95. Yesavage, J. A. and T. L. Rose. Semantic Elaboration and the Method of Loci: A New Trip for Old Learners. *Experimental Aging Research* 10: 155–160 (1984). See also Anschutz, L., C. J. Camp, R. P. Markley, and J. J. Kramer. Maintenance and Generalization of Mnemonics for Grocery Shopping by Older Adults. *Experimental Aging Research* 11:157–160 (1985).

96. Higbee, K. L. *Op. cit.*

97. Paris J. *Op. cit.*

98. Edelman, G. *Brilliant Air, Brilliant Fire: On the Matter of the Mind.* New York: Basic Books, 1992.

99. Barclay, C. R. Schematization of Autobiographical Memory. In D. C. Rubin, ed. *Autobiographical Memory.* Cambridge: Cambridge University Press, 1986. 82–99.

100. Miller, G. A. *Op. cit.*

101. Luria, A. R. *The Mind of a Mnemonist.* Cambridge: Harvard University Press, 1968.

102. Schacter, D. L. *Op. cit.*

103. Biederman, I., E. E. Cooper, P. W. Fox, and R. S. Mahadevan. Unexceptional Spatial Memory in an Exceptional Memorist.

Journal of Experimental Psychology, Learning, Memory, and Cognition 18(3): 654–657 (1992).

104. Algernon Charles Swinburne. *An Interlude,* st. 14.

105. Higbee, K. L. *Op. cit.*

106. Sommer, W., E. Komoss, and S. R. Schweinberger. Differential Localization of Brain System Subserving Memory for Names and Faces in Normal Subjects with Event-related Potentials. *Electroencephalography and Clinical Neurophysiology* 102(3): 192–199 (1997).

107. Sommer, W., A. Heinz, H. Leuthold, J. Matt, and S. R. Schweinberger. Metamemory, Distinctiveness, and Event-related Potentials in Recognition Memory for Faces. *Memory and Cognition* 23(1): 1–11 (1995).

108. Craigie, M., and J. R. Hanley. Putting Faces to Names. *British Journal of Psychology* 88 (Pt. 1)(-EM-): 157–171 (1977).

109. Bazargan, M. and A. R. Barbre. The Effects of Depression, Health Status, and Stressful Life-events on Self-reported Memory Problems Among Aged Blacks. *International Journal of Aging and Human Development* 38(4): 351–362 (1994).

110. Secrets of Good Health for Men and Women in their 40s, their 50s, and 60 +. Wisdom from the Nation's Top Doctors. *Bottom Line Personal* 18(21): 9–10 (1 November 1997).

111. *Ibid.*

112. *Ibid.*

113. Gray, G. E. Nutrition and Dementia. *Journal of the American Dietetic Association* 89(12): 1795–1802 (1989).

114. *Ibid.*

115. Mathew, R. J. and W. H. Wilson. Substance Abuse and Cerebral Blood Flow. *American Journal of Psychiatry* 148(3): 292–305 (1991).

116. Information from the research website of Park Research Lab, *http://www.isr.urmich.edu/rcgd/parklab/research/alcohol. html* [no period].

117. Maylor, E. A., and P. M. Rabbitt. Effect of Alcohol on Rate of Forgetting. *Psychopharmacology (Berlin)* 91(2): 230–235 (1987).

118. Martin, D. and H. S. Swartzwelder. Ethanol Inhibits Release of Excitatory Amino Acids from Slices of Hippocampal Area CA1. *European Journal of Pharmacology* 219(3): 469–472 (4 September 1992).

119. Young Brains Damaged by Alcohol. *Ivanhoe's Medical Breakthroughs.* News Flash 96, Nov. 18–24, 1997. Located at *http://www.ivanhoe.com/docs/backissues/newsflash 96november18to24.html* [no period].

120. Swartzwelder, H. S., K. L. Farr, W. A. Wilson, and D. D. Savage. Prenatal Exposure to Ethanol Decreases Physiological Plasticity in the Hippocampus of the Adult Rat. *Alcohol* 5(2): 121–124 (1988).

121. Walker, M. D. and R. H. Casdorph. *Toxic Metal Syndrome.* Garden City Park, N.Y.: Avery Publications Group, 1995.

122. Willers, S., R. Attewell, I. Bensyrd, A. Schutz, G. Skarping, and M. Vahter. Exposure to Environmental Tobacco Smoke in the Household and Urinary Cotinine Excretion, Heavy Metals Retention, and Lung Function. *Archives of Environmental Health* 47(5): 357–363 (1992). See also Landsberger, S., S. Larson, and D. Wu. Determination of Airborne Cadmium in Environmental Tobacco Smoke by Instrumental Neutron Activation Analysis with a Compton Suppression System. *Annals of Chemistry* 65(11): 1506–1509 (1993).

123. Shaham, J., A. Meltzer, R. Ashkenzai, and J. Ribak. Biological Monitoring of Exposure to Cadmium, a Human Carcinogen, as a Result of Active and Passive Smoking. *Journal of Occupational and Environmental Medicine* 38(12): 1220–1228 (1996).

124. Preston, A. M. Cigarette Smoking—Nutritional Implications. *Progress in Food and Nutrition Science* 15(4): 183–217 (1991).

125. Breslau, N., E. L. Peterson, L. R. Schultz, H. D. Chilcoat, and P. Andreski. Major Depression and Stages of Smoking. A Longitudinal Investigation. *Archives of General Psychiatry* 55(2): 161–166 (1998).

126. Batel, P., F. Pessione, C. Maitre, and B. Rueff. Relationship Between Alcohol and Tobacco Dependencies Among Alcoholics Who Smoke, *Addiction* 90(7): 977–980 (1995).

127. Marks, J. L., E. M. Hill, C. S. Pomerleau, S. A. Mudd, F. C. Blow. Nicotine Dependence and Withdrawal in Alcoholic and Nonalcoholic Ever-smokers. *Journal of Substance Abuse and Treatment* 14(6): 521–527 (1997).

128. Huseman, C. A., M. M. Varma, and C. R. Angle. Neuroendocrine Effects of Toxic and Low Blood Lead Levels in Children. *Pediatrics* 90(2, Pt. 1): 186–189 (1992).

129. Morrow, L. A., S. R. Steinhauer, R. Condray, and M. Hodgson. Neuropsychological Performance of Journeymen Painters Under Acute Solvent Exposure and Exposure-free Conditions. *Journal of the International Neuropsychological Society* 3: 269–275 (1997).

130. Brown, K. S. Risky Business. *Living Fit* 4(5): 82–86, 125 (April 1998).

131. Boosting Your Immune System. *University of California at Berkeley Wellness Letter* 10(1): 4–5 (October 1993).

132. Mietto, L., Boarato, E., G. Toffano, and A. Bruni. Lysophosphatidylserine-dependent Interaction Between Rat Leukocytes and Mast Cells. *Biochimica et Biophysica Acta* 930(2): 145–153 (1987).

133. Samson, J. C. *Op. cit.*

134. Perrig, W. J., P. Perrig, and H. B. Stähelin. The Relation Between Antioxidants and Memory Performance in the Old and Very Old. *Journal of the American Geriatrics Society* 45(6): 718–724 (1997).

135. Walsh, J. Low Fat, No Fat, Some Fat . . . High Fat? Type of

Fat, Not Amount, May Be Key. *Environmental Nutrition* 21(4): 1, 6 (April 1998).

136. Simopoulos, A. P. Preventing Illness with Fish or Fish Oil. *Bottom Line Health* 12(4): 3–4 (April 1998).

137. Rogers, P. J., J. Tonkiss, and J. L. Smart. Incidental Learning Is Impaired During Early-life Undernutrition. *Developmental Psychobiology* 19(2): 113–124 (1986).

138. Yokogoshi, H., and M. Nomura. Effect of Amino Acid Supplementation to a Low-protein Diet on Brain Neurotransmitters and Memory-learning Ability of Rats. *Physiology and Behavior* 50(6): 1227–1232 (1991).

139. Green, M. W., P. J. Rogers, N. A. Elliman, and S. J. Gatenby. Impairment of Cognitive Performance Associated with Dieting and High Levels of Dietary Restraint. *Physiology and Behavior* 55(3): 447–452 (1994).

140. Means, L. W., J. L. Higgins, T. J. Fernandez. Mid-life Onset of Dietary Restriction Extends Life and Prolongs Cognitive Functioning. *Physiology and Behavior* 54(3): 503–508 (1993).

141. Walford, R. L. Calorie Restriction. The Aggressive Anti-aging Plan. *Bottom Line Health* 12(2): 13–14 (February 1998).

142. Kidd, P. M. *Op. cit.*

143. Gray, G. E. *Op. cit.*

144. Larson, E. B., W. A. Kukull, D. Buchner, and B. V. Reifler. Adverse Drug Reactions Associated with Global Cognitive Impairment in Elderly Persons. *Annals of Internal Medicine* 107(2): 169–173 (1987).

145. Bowen, J. D. and E. B. Larson. Drug-induced Cognitive Impairment. Defining the Problem and Finding Solutions. *Drugs and Aging* 3(4): 349–357 (1993).

146. Fogler, J. and L. Stern. *Improving Your Memory,* Rev. ed. Baltimore: The Johns Hopkins University Press, 1994.

147. Monmaney, T. Medications Kill 100,000 Annually, Study Says. *Los Angeles Times,* 5 April 1998, A1, A-22.

148. Rauscher, F. H., G. L. Shaw, and K. N. Ky. Listening to Mozart Enhances Special-temporal Reasoning: Towards a Neurophysiological Basis. *Neuroscience Letters* 185(1): 44–47 (1995).

149. Sarnthein, J., A. von Stein, P. Rappelsberger, H. Petsche, F. H. Rauscher, and G. L. Shaw. Persistent Patterns of Brain Activity: An EEG Coherence Study of the Positive Effect of Music on Spatial-temporal Reasoning. *Neurological Research* 19(2): 107–116 (1997).

150. Rauscher, F. H., G. L. Shaw, L. J. Levine, E. L. Wright, W. R. Dennis, and R. L. Newcomb. Music Training Causes Long-term Enhancement of Preschool Children's Spatial-temporal Reasoning. *Neurological Research* 19(1): 2–8 (1997).

151. Rideout, B. E. and J. Taylor. Enhanced Spatial Performance Following 10 Minutes Exposure to Music: A Replication. *Perceptual Motor Skills* 85(1): 112–114 (1997).

152. Campbell, D. *The Mozart Effect.* New York: Avon Books, 1997.

153. Rideout, B. E., and J. Taylor. *Op. cit.*

154. Cockerton, T., S. Moore, and D. Norman. Cognitive Test Performance and Background Music. *Perceptual Motor Skills* 84(3, Pt. 2): 1435–1438 (1997).

155. Campbell, D. *Op. cit.*

156. Nittono, H. Background Instrumental Music and Serial Recall. *Perceptual Motor Skills* 84(3, Pt. 2): 1307–1313 (1997).

157. Campbell, *Op. cit.*

158. *Ibid.*

159. Heitz, L., T. Symreng, and F. L. Scamman. Effect of Music Therapy in the Post-anesthesia Care Unit: A Nursing Intervention. *Journal of Post Anesthesia Nursing* 7(1): 22–31 (1992).

160. Ostrander, S. and L. Schroeder. *Superlearning 2000*. New York: Delacorte Press, 1994.

161. French studies by A. Lancry cited in Leconte, P. Chronobiological Rhythm Constraints of Memory Processes. In Derouesné, C., D. Guez, and J. P. Poirir, eds. *Memory and Aging*. Amsterdam: Elsevier Science Publishers, 1989. 1–6.

162. Tyler, V. Herbs and Medicines May Not Mix. *Bottom Line Personal* 19(1): 16 (1 January 1998).

163. Pritz-Hohmeier, S., T. I. Chao, J. Krenzlin, and A. Reichenbach. Effect of In Vivo Application of the *Ginkgo biloba* Extract EGb 761 (Rokan) on the Susceptibility of Mammalian Retinal Cells to Proteolytic Enzymes. *Ophthalmic Research* 26(2): 80–86 (1994).

164. Apaydin, C., Y. Oguz, A. Agar, P. Yargicoglu, N. Demir, and G. Aksu. Visual Evoked Potentials and Optic Nerve Histopathology in Normal and Diabetic Rats and Effect of *Ginkgo biloba* Extract. *Acta Ophthalmologica (Copenhagen)* 71(5): 623–628 (1993).

165. Wada, K., K. Sasaki, K. Miura, M. Yagi, Y. Kubota, T. Matsumoto, and M. Haga. Isolation of Bilobalide and Ginkgolide A from *Ginkgo biloba L.* Shorten the Sleeping Time Induced in Mice by Anesthetics, *Biological and Pharmaceutical Bulletin* 16(2): 210–212 (1993).

166. Stoll, S., K. Scheuer, O. Pohl, and W. E. Muller. *Ginkgo biloba* Extract (EGb 761) Independently Improves Changes in Passive Avoidance Learning and Brain Membrane Fluidity in the Aging Mouse. *Pharmacopsychiatry* 29(4): 144–149 (1996).

167. Winter, J. C. The Effects of an Extract of *Ginkgo biloba*, EGB 761, on Cognitive Behavior and Longevity in the Rat. *Physiology and Behavior* 63(3): 425–433 (1998).

168. Le Bars, P. L., M. M. Katz, N. Berman, T. M. Itil, A. M. Freedman, and A. F. Schatzberg. A Placebo-controlled, Double-blind, Randomized Trial of an Extract of *Ginkgo biloba*

for Dementia. North American EGb Study Group. *Journal of the American Medical Association* 278(16): 1327–1332 (22 October 1997).

169. *Ibid.*

170. Allain, H., P. Raoul, A. Lieury, F. LeCoz, J. M. Gandon, and P. d'Arbigny. Effect of Two Doses of *Ginkgo biloba* Extract (EGb 761) on the Dual-coding Test in Elderly Subjects. *Clinical Therapies* 15(3): 549–558 (1993).

171. Grassel, E. [Effect of *Ginkgo-biloba* Extract on Mental Performance. Double-blind Study Using Computerized Measurement Conditions in Patients with Cerebral Insufficiency.] Published in German; English summary. *Fortschritte der Medizin* 110(5): 73–76 (20 February 1992).

172. Blumenthal, M. Canada Approves Ginkgo for Food Use. *HerbalGram*, Summer 1995. Taken from the Internet at *www.healthy.net/library/journals/HerbalGram/1995/summer/legalreg/ginkgo.htm* [no period].

173. Sticher, O. *Ginkgo biloba:* A Modern Phytomedicine. *Vierteljahrsschrift der Naturforschenden Gesellschaft in Zeurich* 138(3): 125–168 (1993).

174. Weiner, M. A. and J. Weiner. *Herbs that Heal.* Mill Valley, Calif.: Quantum Books, 1994.

175. Environmental Nutrition. *The Newsletter of Food, Nutrition & Health* 21(3): 8 (March 1988).

176. Meck, W. H., R. A. Smith, and C. L. Williams. Pre- and Postnatal Choline Supplementation Produces Long-term Facilitation of Spatial Memory. *Developmental Psychobiology* 21(4): 339–353 (1988).

177. Masuda, Y., T. Kokubu, M. Yamashita, H. Ikeda, and S. Inoue. EGG Phosphatidylcholine Combined with Vitamin B_{12} Improved Memory Impairment Following Lesioning of Nucleus Basalis in Rats. *Life Sciences* 62(9): 813–822 (1998).

178. Alvarez, X. A., M. Laredo, D. Corzo, L. Fernandez-Novoa,

R. Mouzo, J. E. Perea, D. Daniele, and R. Cacabelos. Citocoline Improves Memory Performance in Elderly Subjects. *Methods and Findings in Experimental and Clinical Pharmacology* 19(3): 201–210 (1997).

179. Ladd, S. L., S. A. Sommer, S. LaBerge, and W. Toscano. Effect of Phosphatidylcholine on Explicit Memory. *Clinical Neuropharmacology* 16(6): 540–549 (1993).

180. Winter, A. and R. Winter. *Eat Right, Be Bright.* New York: St. Martin's Press, 1988.

181. Carper, J. *Food—Your Miracle Medicine.* New York: HarperPerennial, 1993.

182. Potter, B. A. and S. Orfali. *Op. cit.*

183. Vitamins: Charting Your Course. *University of California at Berkeley Wellness Letter.* 10(4): 4–5 (January 1994).

184. Balch, J. F. and P. A. Balch. *Prescription for Natural Healing.* 2d ed. Garden City Park, N.Y.: Avery Publishing Group, 1997.

185. Winter, A. and R. Winter. *Op. cit.*

186. Balch, J. F. and P. A. Balch. *Op. cit.*

187. *Ibid.*

188. Wild, R., ed. *The Complete Book of Natural and Medicinal Cures.* Emmaus, PA: Rodale Press, 1994.

189. Winter, A. and R. Winter. *Op. cit.*

190. *Ibid.*

191. Wild, R., ed. *Op. cit.*

192. Winter, A. and R. Winter. *Op. cit.*

193. Hoffer, A. and Walker, M. *Op. cit.*

194. Winter, A. and R. Winter. *Op. cit.*

195. Balch, J. F. and P. A. Balch. *Op. cit.*

196. Winter, A. and R. Winter. *Op. cit.*

197. Dean, W. and J. Morgenthaler. *Smart Drugs & Nutrients.* Santa Cruz, California: B & J Publications, 1990.

198. Balch, J. F. and P. A. Balch. *Op. cit.*

199. Deijan, J. B., E. J. van der Beek, J. F. Orlebeke, and H. van

den Berg. Vitamin B_6 Supplementation in Elderly Men: Effects on Mood, Memory, Performance and Mental Effort. *Psychopharmacology (Berlin)* 109(4): 489–496 (1992).

200. Winter, A. and R. Winter. *Op. cit.*

201. Dean, W. and J. Morgenthaler. *Op. cit.*

202. Winter, A. and R. Winter. *Op. cit.*

203. Balch, J. G. and P. A. Balch. *Op. cit.*

204. Winter, A. and R. Winter. *Op. cit.*

205. Socci, D. J., B. M. Crandall, and G. W. Arendash. Chronic Antioxidant Treatment Improves the Cognitive Performance of Aged Rats. *Brain Research* 693(1–2): 88–94 (25 September 1995).

206. Wild, R., ed. *Op. cit.*

207. Jama, J. W., L. J. Launer, J. C. Witteman, J. H. den Breeijen, M. M. Breteler, D. E. Grobbee, and A. Hofman. Dietary Antioxidants and Cognitive Function in a Population-based Sample of Older Persons. The Rotterdam Study. *American Journal of Epidemiology* 144(3): 275–280 (1966).

208. Balch, J. F. and P. A. Balch. *Op. cit.*

209. Wild, R., ed. *Op. cit.*

210. de Angelis, L. and C. Furlan. The Effects of Ascorbic Acid and Oxiracetam on Scopolamine-induced Amnesia in a Habituation Test in Aged Mice. *Neurobiology of Learning and Memory* 64(2): 119–124 (1995).

211. Balch, J. F. and P. A. Balch. *Op. cit.*

212. *Ibid.*

213. *Ibid.*

214. Anonymous. Wellness Made Easy column. *University of California at Berkeley Wellness Letter.* 14(8): 8 (May 1998).

215. Hoffer, A. and M. Walker. *Op. cit.*

216. Winter, A. and R. Winter. *Op. cit.*

217. *Ibid.*

218. Wild, R., ed. *Op. cit.*

219. Balch, J. F. and P. A. Balch. *Op. cit.*

220. *Ibid.*

221. *Ibid.*

222. Weiner, M. A. *Reducing the Risk of Alzheimer's.* New York: Stein and Day, 1987.

223. Gottlieb, B., ed.-in-chief. *The Complete Book of Natural & Medicinal Cures.* Emmaus, Pa.: Rodale Press, 1994.

224. Halas, E. S., M. J. Eberhardt, M. A. Diers, and H. H. Sandstead. Learning and Memory Impairment in Adult Rats Due to Severe Zinc Deficiency During Lactation. *Physiological Behavior* 30(3): 371–381 (1983). See also Halas, E. S., C. D. Hunt, and M. J. Eberhardt. Learning and Memory Disabilities in Young Adult Rats from Mildly Zinc Deficient Dams. *Physiological Behavior* 37(3): 451–458 (1986).

225. Oldereid, N. B., Y. Thomassen, and K. Purvis. Seminal Plasma Lead, Cadmium and Zinc in Relation to Tobacco Consumption. *International Journal of Andrology* 17(1): 24–28 (1994).

226. Winter, A. and R. Winter. *Op. cit.*

227. Calcium Trap. *Bottom Line Health* 12(4): 13 (April 1998).

228. Wild, R., ed. *Op. cit.*

229. Penland, J. G. Dietary Boron, Brain Function, and Cognitive Performanc *Environmental Health Perspectives* 102 (Suppl. 7): 65–72 (1994).

230. Balch, J. F. and P. A. Balch. *Op. cit.*

231. *Ibid.*

232. *Ibid.*

233. Wild, R., ed. *Op. cit.*

234. Potter, B. A. and S. Orfali. *Op. cit.*

235. Wild, R., ed. *Op. cit.*

236. Food as Medicine. *Women's Health Watch* 5(8): 4–5 (April 1998).

237. Cavanaugh, J. C., J. G. Grady, and M. Perlmutter. Forgetting and Use of Memory Aids in 20- to 70-Year-Olds' Everyday

Life. *International Journal of Aging and Human Development* 17: 113–22 (1983).

238. Higbee, K. L. *Op. cit.*

239. Lordi, B., P. Protais, D. Mellier, and J. Caston. Acute Stress in Pregnant Rats: Effects on Growth Rate, Learning, and Memory Capabilities in the Offspring. *Physiology and Behavior* 62(5): 1087–1092 (1997).

240. Magarinos, A. M., J. M. Verdugo, and B. S. McEwen. Chronic Stress Alters Synaptic Terminal Structure in Hippocampus. *Proceedings of the National Academy of Sciences of the United States of America* 94(25): 14002–14008 (1997).

241. Lupien, S. J., S. Gaudreau, B. M. Tchiteya, F. Maheu, S. Sharma, N. P. Nair, R. L. Hauger, B. S. McEwen, and M. J. Meaney. Stress-induced Declarative Memory Impairment in Healthy Elderly Subjects: Relationship to Cortisol Reactivity. *Journal of Clinical Endocrinology and Metabolism* 82(7): 2070–2075 (1997).

242. Campbell, D. *Op. cit.*

243. Healing Column. *Bottom Line Tomorrow.* 6(1): 15 (January 1998).

244. Pelletier, K. R. *Ibid.* (see #84)

245. Coren, Stanley. *Sleep Thieves: An Eye-opening Exploration into the Science and Mysteries of Sleep.* Monroe, La.: The Active Record Free Press, 1996.

246. *Macbeth* 2.2.39.

247. Thomson, S. A. *Cloud Nine. A Dreamer's Dictionary.* New York: Avon Books, 1994.

248. Anonymous. Nourishing Sleep: Meeting Changing Needs. *The Johns Hopkins Medical Letter. Health After 50.* 5(8): 4–6 (October 1993).

249. Sobel, D. and Ornstein, R., eds. Exercise Improves Sleep. *Mind/Body Health Newsletter* 6(1): 1 (1997).

250. Cooper, K. Dr. Ken Cooper Tells How to Get Back in Shape. *Bottom Line Personal* 19(6): 9–11 (15 March 1988).

251. Butler, K. and L. Rayner. *The New Handbook of Health and Preventive Medicine.* Buffalo: N.Y.: Prometheus Books, 1990.

252. Water Workouts: A Low-Impact Way to Stay Fit. *Harvard Health Letter* 23(4): 6–7 (February 1998).

253. You can contact the U.S. Water Fitness Association at P.O. Box 3279, Boynton Beach, FL 33424, tel. (561) 732-9908.

254. Dawe, D. and R. Moore-Orr. Low-intensity, Range-of-motion Exercise: Invaluable Nursing Care for Elderly Patients. *Journal of Advanced Nursing* 21(4): 675–681 (1995).

255. Williams, P. and S. R. Lord. Effects of Group Exercise on Cognitive Functioning and Mood in Older Women. *Australian and New Zealand Journal of Public Health* 21(1): 45–52 (1997).

256. Slaven, L. and C. Lee. Mood and Symptom Reporting Among Middle-aged Women: The Relationship Between Menopausal Status, Hormone Replacement Therapy, and Exercise Participation. *Health Psychology* 16(3): 203–208 (1997).

257. Satoh, T., I. Sakurai, K. Miyagi, Y. Hohshaku. Walking Exercise and Improved Neuropsychological Functioning in Elderly Patients with Cardiac Disease. *Journal of Internal Medicine* 238(5): 423–428 (1995).

258. Breitner, J. C. S., J. M. Silverman, R. C. Mohs, and K. C. Davis. Familiar Aggregation of Alzheimer's Disease: Comparison of Risk Among Relatives of Early and Late Onset Causes, and Among Male and Female Relatives in Successive Generations. *Neurology* 38: 207–212 (1988).

259. Crook, Thomas H. III, Diagnosis and Treatment of Memory Loss in Older Patients Who Are Not Demented. Treatment and Care in Old Age, *Psychiatry* 95–111 (1993).

260. *Advances in Alzheimer's Disease Research.* La Jolla: The Salk Institute for Biological Studies, 1996.

261. Snowdon, D. A., S. J. Kemper, J. A. Mortimer, L. H. Greiner,

D. R. Wekstein, and W. R. Markesbery. Linguistic Ability in Early Life and Cognitive Function and Alzheimer's Disease in Late Life. Findings from the Nun Study. *Journal of the American Medical Association* 275(7): 528–532 (21 February 1996).

262. Genetic Testing and Alzheimer's Disease. *Health News* 4(4): 5 (31 March 1988).

263. Fujishima, M., S. Ibayashi, K. K. Fujii, and S. Mori. Cerebral Blood Flow and Brain Function in Hypertension. *Hypertension Research* 18(2): 111–117 (1995).

264. Waldstein, S. R., S. B. Manuck, C. M. Ryan, and M. F. Muldoon. Neuropsychological Correlates of Hypertension: Review and Methodologic Consideration. *Psychological Bulletin* 110(3): 451–468 (1991).

265. Nakamura-Palacios, E. M., C. K. Caldas, A. Fiorina, K. D. Chagas, K. N. Chagas, and E. C. Vazquez. Deficits of Spatial Learning and Working Memory in Spontaneously Hypertensive Rats. *Behavioral Brain Research* 74(1–2): 217–227 (1996). See also: Meneses, A., C. Castillo, M. Ibarra, and E. Hong. Effects of Aging and Hypertension on Learning, Memory, and Activity in Rats. *Physiological Behavior* 60(2): 341–345 (1996).

266. Wyss, J. M., G. Fisk, and T. Van Groen. Impaired Learning and Memory in Mature Spontaneously Hypertensive Rats. *Brain Research* 592(1–2): 135–140 (2 October 1992).

267. Launer, L. J., K. Masaki, H. Petrovitch, D. Foley, and R. J. Havlik. The Association Between Midlife Blood Pressure Levels and Late-life Cognitive Function. The Honolulu-Asia Aging Study. *Journal of the American Medical Association* 274(23): 1846–1851 (20 December 1995).

268. Starr, J. M., L. J. Whalley, and I. J. Dreary. The Effects of Antihypertensive Treatment on Cognitive Function: Results from the HOPE Study. *Journal of the American Geriatric Society* 44(4): 411–415 (1996).

269. Kuusisto, J., K. Koivisto, L. Mykkanenm, E. L. Helkala, M. Vanhanen, T. Hanninen, K. Pyorala, P. Riekkinen, and M. Laakso. Essential Hypertension and Cognitive Function. The Role of Hyperinsulinemia. *Hypertension* 22(5): 771–779 (1993).

270. Strassburger, T. L., H. C. Lee, E. M. Daly, J. Szczepanik, J. S. Krasuski, M. J. Mentis, J. A. Salerno, C. DeCarli, M. B. Schapiro, and G. E. Alexander. Interactive Effects of Age and Hypertension on Volumes of Brain Structures. *Stroke* 28(7): 1410–1417 (1997).

271. Elias, P. K., R. B. D'Agostino, M. F. Elias, and P. A. Wolf. Blood Pressure, Hypertension, and Age as Risk Factors for Poor Cognitive Performance. *Experimental Aging Research* 21(4): 393–417 (1995).

272. Thyrum, E. T., J. A. Blumenthal, D. J. Madden, and W. Siegel. Family History of Hypertension Influences Neurobehavioral Function in Hypertensive Patients. *Psychosomatic Medicine* 57(5): 496–500 (1995).

273. Berkow, R., M. H. Beers, and A. J. Fletcher, eds. *The Merck Manual of Medical Information.* Home ed. Whitehouse Station, N.J.: Merck Research Laboratories, 1997.

274. Gray, G. E. *Op. cit.*

275. Zhang, X. L., H. Begleiter, B. Porjesz, and A. Litke. Electrophysiological Evidence of Memory Impairment in Alcoholic Patients. *Biological Psychiatry* 42(12): 1157–1171 (1947).

276. Hendrie, H. C., S. Gao, K. S. Hall, S. L. Hui, and F. W. Unverzagt. The Relationship Between Alcohol Consumption, Cognitive Performance, and Daily Functioning in an Urban Sample of Older Black Americans. *Journal of the American Geriatric Society* 44(10): 1158–1165 (1996).

277. Schacter, D. L. *Op. cit.*

278. Berkow, R., M. H. Beers, and A. J. Fletcher, eds. *Op. cit.*

279. Hoffer, A. and M. Walker. *Op. cit.*

280. Wiegand, L. and C. W. Zwillich. Obstructive Sleep Apnea. *Disease-A-Month* 49(4): 197–252 (1994).

281. Nasser, S. and P. J. Rees. Sleep Apnea: Causes, Consequences, and Treatment. *British Journal of Clinical Practice* 46(1): 39–43 (1992).

282. Wiegand, L. and C. W. Zwillich. *Op. cit.*

283. Dealberto, M. J., N. Pajot, D. Courbon, and A. Aleperovitch. Breathing Disorders During Sleep and Cognitive Performance in an Older Community Sample: The EVA Study. *Journal of the American Geriatric Society* 44(11): 1287–1294 (1996).

284. Berry, D. T., B. A. Phillips, Y. R. Cook, F. A. Schmitt, N. A. Honeycutt, A. A. Arita, and R. S. Allen. Geriatric Sleep Apnea Syndrome: A Preliminary Description. *Journal of the Gerontology* 45(5): M169–M174 (1990).

285. Ragozzino, M. E., K. E. Unick, and P. E. Gold. Hippocampal Acetylcholine Release During Memory Testing in Rats: Augmentation by Glucose. *Proceedings of the National Academy of Science, USA* 93(10): 4693–4698 (14 May 1996).

286. Berkow, R., M. H. Beers, and A. J. Fletcher, eds. *Op. cit.*

287. *Ibid.*

288. Gabrieli, J. D. Memory Systems Analyses of Mnemonic Disorders in Aging and Age-related Diseases. *Proceedings of the National Academy of Science, USA* 93(24): 13534–13540 (1996).

289. Pincus, H. A., T. L. Tanielian, S. C. Marcus, M. Olfson, D. A. Zarin, J. Thompson, and J. Mango Zito. Prescribing Trends in Psychotropic Medications: Primary Care, Psychiatry, and Other Medical Specialties. *Journal of the American Medical Association,* 279(7): 526–531 (18 February 1998).

290. Maggioni, M., G. B. Picotti, G. P. Bondiolotti, A. Panerai, T. Cenacchi, P. Nobile, and F. Brambilla. Effects of Phosphatidylserine Therapy in Geriatric Patients with Depressive Dis-

orders. *Acta Psychiatrica Scandinavica* 81(3): 265–270 (1990).

291. Poitrenaud, J., F. Moy, A. Girousse, Y. Wolmark, and F. Piette. Psychometric Procedures for Analysis of Memory Losses in the Elderly. In Derouesné, C., D. Guez, and J. P. Poirier, eds. *Op. cit.* 173–183.

292. Berkow, R., M. H. Beers, and A. J. Fletcher, eds. *Op. cit.*

293. Vasterling, J. J., K. Bailey, J. I. Constans, and P. B. Sutker. Attention and Memory Dysfunction in Posttraumatic Stress Disorder. *Neuropsychology* 12(1): 125–133 (1998).

294. Bremner, J. D., J. H. Crystal, S. M. Southwick, and D. S. Charney. Functional Neuroanatomical Correlates of the Effects of Stress on Memory. *Journal of Traumatic Stress* 8(4): 527–553 (1995).

295. Jenkins, M. A., P. J. Langlais, D. Delis, and R. Cohen. Learning and Memory in Rape Victims with Posttraumatic Stress Disorder. *American Journal of Psychiatry* 155(2): 278–279 (1998).

296. Lawrie, S. A. Is the Chronic Fatigue Syndrome Best Understood as a Primary Disturbance of the Sense of Effort? An Editorial. *Psychological Medicine* 27: 995–999 (1997).

297. Berkow, R., M. H. Beers, and A. J. Fletcher, eds. *Op. cit.*

298. Lawrie, S. M., D. N. Manders, J. R. Geddes, and A. J. Pelosi. A Population-based Incidence Study of Chronic Fatigue. *Psychological Medicine* 27: 343–353 (1997).

299. Berkow, R., M. H. Beers, and A. J. Fletcher, eds. *Op. cit.*

300. Ried, L. D., R. E. Johnson, and D. A. Gettman. Benzodiazepine Exposure and Functional Status in Older People. *Journal of the American Geriatric Society* 46(1): 71–76 (1998).

301. Sharp, K., P. M. Brindle, M. W. Brown, G. M. Turner. Memory Loss During Pregnancy. *British Journal of Obstetrics and Gynaecology* 100(3): 209–215 (1993).

302. Berkow, R., M. H. Beers, and A. J. Fletcher. *Op. cit.*

303. Information from the research website of Park Research Lab,

http://www.isr.umich.edu/rcgd/parklab/research/fm.html [no period].

304. Sightings Column: Surgery and Memory. *Health News* 4(5): 5 (20 April 1988).

305. Helmstaedter, C., U. Gleissner, M. Di Perna, and C. E. Elger. Relational Verbal Memory Processing in Patients with Temporal Lobe Epilepsy. *Cortex* 33(4): 667–678.

306. Anonymous. Brain Tumor: Better Treatments for an Enigmatic Disease. *Harvard Health Letter* 23(6): 6–7 (April 1998).

307. Berkow, R., M. H. Beers, and A. J. Fletcher, eds. *Op. cit.*

308. Berkow, R., M. H. Beers, and A. J. Fletcher, eds. *Op. cit.*

309. Gould, E., C. S. Woolley, and B. S. McEwen. The Hippocampal Formation: Morphological Changes Induced by Thyroid, Gonadal and Adrenal Hormones. *Psychoneuroendocrinology* 16(1–3): 67–84 (1991).

310. Pavlides, C., A. I. Westlind-Danielsson, H. Nyborg, and B. S. McEwen. Neonatal Hyperthyroidism Disrupts Hippocampal LTP and Spatial Learning. *Experimental Brain Research* 85(3): 559–564 (1991).

311. Berkow, R., M. H. Beers, and A. J. Fletcher, eds. *Op. cit.*

312. Kudrjavcev, T. Neurologic Complication of Thyroid Dysfunction. *Advances in Neurology* 19: 619–636 (1978).

313. Osterweil, D., K. Syndulko, S. N. Cohen, P. D. Pettler-Jennings, J. M. Hershman, J. L. Cummings, W. W. Tourtellotte, and D. H. Solomon. Cognitive Function in Non-demented Older Adults with Hypothyroidism. *Journal of the American Geriatric Society* 40(4): 325–335 (1992).

314. Baldini, I. M., A. Vita, M. C. Mauri, V. Amodei, M. Carrisi, S. Bravin, and L. Cantalamessa. Psychopathological and Cognitive Features in Subclinical Hypothyroidism. *Prog Neuropsychopharmacol Bil. Psychiatry* 21(6): 925–935 (1997).

315. Monzani, F., P. Del Guerra, N. Caraccio, C. A. Pruneti, E.

Pucci, M. Luisi, and L. Baschieri. Subclinical Hypothyroidism: Neurobehavioral Features and Beneficial Effect of L-thyroxine Treatment. *Clinical Investigator* 71(5): 367–371 (1993).

316. Jaeschke, R., G. Guyatt, H. Gerstein, C. Patterson, W. Molloy, D. Cook, S. Harper, L. Griffith, and R. Carbotte. Does Treatment with L-thyroxine Influence Health Status in Middle-aged and Older Adults with Subclinical Hypothyroidism? *Journal of General Internal Medicine* 11(12): 744–749 (1996).

317. Howe, M. L., M. L. Courage. The Emergence and Early Development of Autobiographical Memory. *Psychological Review* 104(3): 499–523 (1997).

318. Kopelman, M. D. Amnesia: Organic and Psychogenic. *British Journal of Psychiatry* 150: 428–442 (1987).

319. Schacter, D. L. *Op. cit.*

320. Kopelman, M. D. *Op. cit.*

321. Berkow, R., M. H. Beers, and A. J. Fletcher, eds. *Op. cit.*

322. Beatty, W. W., D. E. Goodkin, N. Monson, P. A. Beatty, and D. Hertsgaard. Anterograde and Retrograde Amnesia in Patients with Chronic Progressive Multiple Sclerosis. *Archives of Neurology* 45: 611–619 (1988). See also Beatty, W. W., D. E. Goodkin, N. Monson, and P. A. Beatty. Cognitive Disturbances in Patients with Relapsing Remitting Multiple Sclerosis. *Archives of Neurology* 46: 1113–1119 (1989).

323. Rao, S. M., G. J. Leo, L. Bernardin, and F. Unverzagt. Cognitive Dysfunction in Multiple Sclerosis. I: Frequency, Patterns, and Prediction. *Neurology* 41: 685–691 (1991).

324. Paul, R. H., C. R. Blanco, K. A. Hames, and W. W. Beatty. Autobiographical Memory in Multiple Sclerosis. *Journal of the International Neuropsychological Society* 3: 246–251 (1997).

325. Bruner, A. B., A. Joffe, A. K. Duggan, J. F. Casella, and J. Brandt. Randomized Study of Cognitive Effects of Iron

Supplementation in Non-anemic Iron-deficient Adolescent Girls. *Lancet* 348(9033): 992–996 (12 October 1996).

326. *Ibid.*

327. Berkow, R., M. H. Beers, and A. J. Fletcher, eds. *Op. cit.*

328. Huang, C. C. and N. S. Chu. Wilson's disease: Resolution of MRI Lesions Following Long-term Oral Zinc Therapy. *Acta Neurologica Scandinavia* 17(4): 215–218 (1996).

329. Berkow, R., Ed.-in-Chief. *The Merck Manual of Diagnosis and Therapy.* 14th ed. Rahway, N.J.: Merck, Sharp & Dohme Research Laboratories, 1982.

330. Potter, B. A. and S. Orfali. *Op. cit.*

331. Saletu, B., G. Hitzenberger, J. Grunberger, P. Anderer, G. Zylharz, L. Linzmayer, and H. Ramesis. Double-blind, Placebo-controlled, Pharmacokinetic and -dynamic Studies with Two New Formulations of Piracetam (Infusion and Sirup) Under Hypoxia in Man. *International Journal of Clinical Pharmacology and Therapeutics* 33(5): 249–262 (1995).

332. Brandao, F., A. Cadete-Leite, J. P. Andrade, M. D. Madeira, and M. M. Paula-Barbosa. Piracetam Promotes Mossy Fiber Synaptic Reorganization in Rats Withdrawn from Alcohol. *Alcohol* 13(3): 239–249 (1996).

333. Pilch, H., and W. E. Muller. Piracetam Elevates Muscarinic Cholinergic Receptor Density in the Frontal Cortex of Aged But Not of Young Mice. *Psychopharmacology (Berlin)* 94(1): 74–78 (1988).

334. Vernon, M. W. and E. M. Sorkin. Piracetam. An Overview of Its Pharmacological Properties and a Review of Its Therapeutic Use in Senile Cognitive Disorders. *Drugs and Aging* 1(1): 17–35 (1991).

335. Gromov, L. A., V. A. Portniagina, P. I. Sereda, and L. S. Bobkova. [Pharmacologic Analysis of the Free Radical Mechanism of Poisoning-Induced Memory Disorders.] Article in Russian; summary in English. *Patologicheskaia Fiziologiia I Eksperimentalnaia Terapiia* 1: 8–10 (1993).

336. Israel, L., M. Melac, D. Milinkevitch, and G. Dubos. Drug Therapy and Memory Training Programs: A Double-blind Randomized Trial of General Practice Patients with Age-associated Memory Impairment. *International Psychogeriatrics* 6(2): 155–170 (1994).

337. Deberdt, W. Interaction Between Psychological and Pharmacological Treatment in Cognitive Impairment. *Life Sciences* 55(25–26): 2057–2066 (1994).

338. *Ibid.*

339. Dasaeva, L. A. [Effects of Piracetam on Occupationally Significant Functions of Patients with Arterial Hypertension Working Under Conditions of Psychoemotional Stress.] Article in Russian; summary in English. *Meditsina Truda I Promyshlennaia Ekologiia* 10: 26–28 (1995).

340. Vernon, M. W. and E. M. Sorkin. *Op. cit.*

341. Gouliaev, A. H., A. Senning. Piracetam and Other Structurally Related Nootropics. *Brain Research. Brain Research Reviews* 19(2): 180–222 (1994).

342. Flood, J. F., G. E. Smith, and A. Cherkin. Hydergine Enhances Memory in Mice. *Journal of Pharmacology* 16 (Suppl. 3): 39–49 (1985).

343. McConnachie, R. W. The Clinical Assessment of Brain Failure in the Elderly. *Pharmacology* 16 (Suppl. 1): 27–35 (1978).

344. Thienhaus, O. J., B. G. Wheeler, S. Simon, F. P. Zemlan, and J. T. Hartford. A Controlled Double-blind Study of High-dose Dihydroergotoxine Mesylate (Hydergine) in Mild Dementia. *Journal of the American Geriatric Society* 34(3): 219–223 (1987).

345. Balch, J. F. and P. A. Blach. *Op. cit.*

346. Shigenaga, M. K., T. M. Hagen, and B. N. Ames. Oxidative Damage and Mitochondrial Decay in Aging. *Proceedings of the National Academy of Sciences of the United States of America* 91(23): 10771–10778 (8 November 1994).

347. Passeri, M., M. Iannuccelli, G. Ciotti, P. A. Bonati, G. Nolfe, D. Cucinotta. Mental Impairment in Aging: Selection of Patients, Methods of Evaluation and Therapeutic Possibilities of Acetyl-L-carnitine. *International Journal of Clinical Pharmacology Research* 8(5): 367–376 (1988).

348. Passeri, M., D. Cucinotta, P. A. Bonati, M. Iannuccelli, L. Parnetti, and U. Senin. Acetyl-L-carnitine in the Treatment of Mildly Demented Elderly Patients. *International Journal of Clinical Pharmacology Research* 10(1–2): 75–79 (1990).

349. Arrigo, A., R. Casale, M. Buonocore, and C. Ciano. Effects of Acetyl-L-carnitine on Reaction Times in Patients with Cerebrovascular Insufficiency. *International Journal of Clinical Pharmacology Research* 10(1–2): 133–137 (1990).

350. Carta, A., M. Calvani, D. Bravi, and S. N. Bhuachalla. Acetyl-L-carnitine and Alzheimer's Disease: Pharmacological Considerations Beyond the Cholinergic Sphere. *Annals of the New York Academy of Sciences* 695: 324–326 (24 September 1993).

351. Pettegrew, J. W., W. E. Klunk, K. Panchalingam, J. N. Kanfer, and R. J. McClure. Clinical and Neurochemical Effects of Acetyl-L-carnitine in Alzheimer's Disease. *Neurobiology of Aging* 16(1): 1–4 (1995).

352. Rai, G., G. Wright, L. Scott, B. Beston, J. Rest, A. N. Exton-Smith. Double-blind, Placebo Controlled Study of Acetyl-L-carnitine in Patients with Alzheimer's Dementia. *Current Medical Research and Opinion* 11(10): 638–647 (1990).

353. Thal, L. J., A. Carta, W. R. Clarke, S. H. Ferris, R. P. Friedland, R. C. Peterson, J. W. Pettegrew, E. Pfeiffer, M. A. Raskind, M. Sano, M. H. Tuszynski, and R. F. Woolson. A 1-year Multicenter Placebo-controlled Study of Acetyl-L-carnitine in Patients with Alzheimer's Disease. *Neurology* 47(3): 705–711 (1996).

354. Dean, W., J. Morgenthaler, and S. W. Fowkes. *Smart Drugs*

II. The Next Generation. Menlo Park, CA: Health Freedom Publications, 1993.

355. Slotten, H. A., and S. Krekling. Does Melatonin Have an Effect on Cognitive Performance? *Psychoneuroendocrinology* 21(8): 673–680 (1996).

356. Folkard, S., J. Arendt, and M. Clark. Can Melatonin Improve Shift Workers' Tolerance of the Night Shift? Some Preliminary Findings. *Chronobiology International* 10(5): 315–320 (1993).

357. Dean, W., J. Morgenthaler, and S. W. Fowkes. *Op. cit.*

358. Knoll, J. (-)Deprenyl-medication: A Strategy to Modulate the Age-related Decline of the Striatal Dopaminergic System. *Journal of the American Geriatric Society* 40(8): 839–847 (1992).

359. Dean, W., J. Morgenthaler, and S. W. Fowkes. *Op. cit.*

360. Dean, W., J. Morgenthaler, and S. W. Fowkes. *Op. cit.*

361. Stoll, S., U. Hafner, O. Pohl, W. E. Míuller. Age-related Memory Decline and Longevity Under Treatment with Selegiline. *Life Sciences* 55(25–26): 2155–2163 (1994).

362. Marin, D. B., L. M. Bierer, B. A. Lawlor, T. M. Ryan, R. Jacobson, J. Schmeidler, R. C. Mohs, and K. L. Davis. L-deprenyl and Physostigmine for the Treatment of Alzheimer's Disease. *Psychiatry Research* 58(3): 181–189 (1995).

363. Finali, G., M. Piccirilli, C. Oliani, and G. L. Piccinin. Alzheimer-type Dementia and Verbal Memory Performances: Influence of Selegiline Therapy. *Italian Journal of Neurological Sciences* 13(2): 141–148 (1992).

364. Finali, G., M. Piccirilli, C. Oliani, and G. L. Piccinin. L-deprenyl Therapy Improves Verbal Memory in Amnesic Alzheimer Patients. *Clinical Neuropharmacology* 14(6): 523–536 (1991).

365. Tariot, P. N., T. Sunderland, H. Weingartner, D. L. Murphy, J. A. Welkowitz, K. Thompson, and R. M. Cohen. *Psychopharmacology (Berlin)* 91(4): 489–495 (1987).

366. Langley, M. S. and E. M. Sorkin. Nimodipine. A Review of Its Pharmacodynamic and Pharmacokinetic Properties, and Therapeutic Potential in Cerebrovascular Disease. *Drugs* 37(5): 669–699 (1989).

367. Levy, A., R. M. Kong, M. J. Stillman, B. Shukitt-Hale, T. Kadar, T. M. Rauch, and H. R. Lieberman. Nimodipine Improves Spatial Working Memory and Elevates Hippocampal Acetylcholine in Young Rats. *Pharmacology, Biochemistry and Behavior* 39(3): 781–786 (1991).

368. Ban, T. A., L. Morey, E. Aguglia, O. Azzarelli, F. Balsano, V. Marigliano, N. Caglieris, M. Sterlicchio, A. Cupurso, N. A. Tomasi, et al. *Progress in Neuro-psychopharmacology and Biological Psychiatry* 14(4): 525–551 (1990).

369. Bennett, T. L. *Brain and Behavior.* Monterey, CA: Brooks/ Cole Publishing Co., 1977.

370. Manton, K. G. and E. Stallard. Longevity in the United States, Age and Sex-specific Evidence on Life Span Limits from Mortality Patterns 1960–1990. *Journals of Gerontology, Series A, Biological Sciences and Medical Sciences* 51(5): B362–375 (1996).

371. Information from the research website of Park Research Lab, *http://www.isr.umich.edu/rcgd/parklab/research/context.html* [no period].

372. Information from the research website of Park Research Lab, *http://www.isr.umich.edu/rcgd/parklab/research/culture.html* [no period].

373. Information from the research website of Park Research Lab, *http://www.isr.umich.edu/rcgd/parklab/research/attention. html* [no period].

374. Information from the research website of Park Research Lab, *http://www.isr.umich.edu/rcgd/parklab/research/alcohol. html* [no period].

375. Information from the research website of Park Research Lab,

http://www.isr.umich.edu/rcgd/parklab/research/stereotype.
html [no period].

376. Buckner, R. L. and W. Koutstaal. Functional Neuroimaging Studies of Encoding, Priming, and Explicit Memory Retrieval. *Proceedings of the National Academy of Sciences* 95(3): 891–898 (3 February 1998).

377. *Advances in Brain Research.* La Jolla: The Salk Institute for Biological Studies, 1996.

378. *Advances in Alzheimer's Disease Research. Op. cit.*

379. Martinez-Serrano, A., W. Fischer, S. Söderström, T. Ebendal, and A. Björkland. *Proceedings of the National Academy of Sciences of the United States of America* 93(13): 6355–6360 (25 June 1996).

380. Paton, J. A. and F. N. Nottebohm. Neurons Generated in the Adult Brain are Recruited into Functional Circuits. *Science* 225(4666): 1046–1048 (7 September 1984).

381. Research News. *Science* 224: 1325–1326 (1984).

382. Gould, E., P. Tanapat, B. S. McEwen, F. Flügge, and E. Fuchs. Proliferation of Granule Cell Precursors in the Dentate Gyrus of Adult Monkeys Is Diminished by Stress. *Proceedings of the National Academy of Sciences of the United States of America* 95(6): 3168–3171 (17 March 1998).

383. Herlitz, A., L. G. Nilsson, and L. Backman. *Memory and Cognition* 25(6), 801–811 (1997).

384. Sherwin, B. B. Estrogen and Cognitive Functioning in Women. *Proceedings of the Society for Experimental Biology and Medicine* 217(1): 17–22 (1998).

385. Fink, G., B. E. Sumner, R. Rosie, O. Grace, and J. P. Quinn. Estrogen Control of Central Neurotransmission: Effect on Mood, Mental State, and Memory. *Cellular and Molecular Neurobiology* 16(3): 325–344 (1996).

386. *Ibid.*

387. Kawas, C., S. Resnick, A. Morrison, R. Brookmeyer, M. Corrada, A. Zonderman, C. Bacal, D. D. Lingle, and E. Metter.

A Prospective Study of Estrogen Replacement Therapy and the Risk of Developing Alzheimer's Disease: The Baltimore Longitudinal Study of Aging. *Neurology* 48(6): 1517–1521 (1997).

388. Resnick, S. M., E. J. Metter, and A. B. Zonderman. Estrogen Replacement Therapy and Longitudinal Decline in Visual Memory. A Possible Protective Effect? *Neurology* 49(6): 1491–1497 (1997).

389. Haskell, S. G., E. D. Richardson, and R. I. Horwitz. The Effect of Estrogen Replacement Therapy on Cognitive Function in Women: A Critical Review of the Literature. *Journal of Clinical Epidemiology* 59(11): 1249–1264 (1997).

390. Yaffe, K., G. Sawaya, I. Lieberburg, and D. Grady. Estrogen Therapy in Postmenopausal Women: Effects on Cognitive Function and Dementia. *Journal of the American Medical Association* 279(9): 688–695 (4 March 1998).

391. Burke, Edmund R. PS: An Answer to Intense Training. *Nutrition Science News* 3 (5): 252–253 (May 1998).

392. Monteleone, P., et al. "Effects of phosphatidylserine on the neuroendocrine response to physical response in humans," *Neuroendocrinology*, 52:243–48, 1990.

393. Monteleone, P., et al. "Blunting by chronic phosphatidylserine administration of the stress-induced activation of the hypothalamo-pituitary-adrenal axis in healthy men," *European Journal of Clinical Pharmacology*, 43:385–88, 1992.

394. Fahey, T.D., and Pearl, M.S. "The hormonal and perceptive effects of phosphatidylserine administration during two weeks of restrictive exercise-induced overtraining," *Biology of Sport*, 15 (3), 1998: 135–144.

GLOSSARY

Absentmindedness   When a person intends to perform one action but unintentionally does another.

Acetylcholine (ACh)   A neurotransmitter that plays an important role in learning, concentration, and memory processes. It is produced by a complex chemical process using acetate and choline molecules. Neurons that release ACh are called cholinergic neurons (see *cholinergic* and also *adrenergic*). After being used, acetylcholine is broken down again into acetate and choline by an enzyme called acetylcholinesterase or AChE.

Action potential   The all-or-none discharge, or nerve impulse, that travels down the axon of a neuron.

Adrenergic   Activated or transmitted by the hormone epinephrine, which is released predominantly in response to low blood sugar. The term applies to sympathetic nerve fibers, which secrete sympathin at a synapse when a nerve impulse passes.

Adrenocorticotrophic hormone (ACTH)   A hormone produced by the adrenal glands that in small doses enhances learning.

Age-associated memory impairment (AAMI)   A term now being phased out that refers to a decline in short-term memory that sometimes accompanies aging, and, in most cases, does not progress to other cognitive impairments such as Alzheimer's disease. It is being replaced by the term *age-related cognitive decline (ARCD)*.

Age-related cognitive decline (ARCD)   A condition that typically occurs in a person 45 years or older and refers to a noticeable decrease in mental performance with no detectable disease that can account for the cognitive loss.

Alzheimer's disease The most common cause of dementia among older people. Typically this progressive, irreversible disorder leads to an obvious loss in short-term and long-term memory, personality changes, and impairment of judgment.

Amnesia Loss of memory due to injury to the brain or to disease.

Amygdala A group of nuclei lying within the anterior medial portion of each temporal lobe of the brain. Comprising part of the limbic system, they are involved in forming long-term memories.

Anterograde amnesia Difficulty learning and remembering new information after brain trauma.

Antioxidants Substances that block or inhibit destructive oxidation reactions, thus preventing the formation of free radicals, or that, after their formation, deactivate them.

ApolipoproteinE gene One form of this gene produces the protein apolipoprotein E4, which occurs more often in people with Alzheimer's disease. The other two forms of the gene, apoE2 and apoE3, may protect against the disease.

Atrophy A wasting away of a tissue or organ.

Axon The long, tube-like extension of a neuron, which transmits outgoing signals away from the cell body to other cells.

Basal ganglia A collection of neurons at the base of the cerebrum.

Beta-amyloid A protein found in dense deposits that form the core of neuritic plaques in Alzheimer's disease.

Beta-blocker A drug used for heart disorders and hypertension that combines with and blocks the activity of a beta receptor and can contribute to memory impairment.

Beta-endorphin A natural opiate released in the brain during stress and pain, affecting memory. Technically not a neurotransmitter, its effects are similar. In general, endorphins stimulate interest, focus, and concentration (see also *endorphins*).

Biosynthesis   The formation or production of a compound from its separate constituents by a living organism.

Blood-brain barrier   A group of mechanisms that work to keep some substances, particularly harmful ones, in the bloodstream and to prevent them from passing out of the blood vessels and entering cells in the brain.

Brain   The collection of nervous and supporting tissue within the skull. The brain and spinal cord together comprise the central nervous system.

Brainstem   The first part of the brain formed, sometimes called the "reptilian brain," it determines our level of alertness and handles automatic bodily functions.

Calcium-channel blocker   A drug that stops calcium from entering cells and is frequently used in the treatment of heart disease and hypertension.

CAT scan   See *Computerized Axial Tomography (CAT scan)*.

Catecholamine   A class of molecules that include the neurotransmitters dopamine, epinephrine, and norepinephrine.

Cell   The smallest unit of a living organism that is capable of functioning independently. Cells consist of a nucleus, cytoplasm, and a cell membrane.

Cellular membrane   The outer boundary of a cell, which is comprised of fats (lipids) and proteins. The membrane controls the flow of substances into and out of the cell.

Cerebellum   That part of the brain that controls movement and stores memory related to movement. Also called the hindbrain.

Cerebral cortex   The outer layer of gray material of the brain and the part of the brain most involved in learning, language, and reasoning. Literally, cortex means bark; the cortex covers the hemispheres of the brain much as bark covers the trunk of a tree.

Cerebrum   In higher mammals, it is the expanded and main portion of the brain, consisting of two hemispheres united by a large bundle of nerve fibers called the corpus callosum. It is considered to be the seat of conscious mental processes.

Cholinergic   Pertaining to choline (acetylcholine), the cholinergic system includes the neurons that release acetylcholine and the neurons and proteins that are stimulated or activated by acetylcholine, i.e., the parasympathetic nerve endings. Cholinesterase hydrolizes (breaks down) acetylcholine into choline and acetic acid.

Cognitive functions   A term lumping all aspects of thinking, perceiving, and remembering.

Computerized axial tomography (CAT scan)   Essentially a computer-enhanced X ray that creates a three-dimensional picture of the body, or part of it. A CAT scan can be used to detect blood clots, brain tumors, shrinkage of the brain, thinning of the neocortex, and the presence of the tangles and plaques typical of Alzheimer's disease.

Consolidation   The physiological process that progressively transforms a temporary memory into a long-term one.

Corpus callosum   A sickle-shaped band of nerve fibers that crosses between the two hemispheres of the brain and interconnects them.

Cortisol   A hormone formed in the adrenal cortex, usually in response to stressful stimuli.

Dementia   A catch-all term for disorders that result in a deterioration of cognitive functions or intellectual abilities, causing confusion, disorientation, and memory loss for recent events, and interfering with a person's normal daily activities and social relationships.

Dendrites   The short, branching extensions of a neuron, which, when stimulated by neurotransmitters, receive impulses ("messages") from other neurons and conduct them toward the cell body.

Depression The emotional state of being sad or down that is often accompanied by difficulty in thinking and concentration and results in lessened memory ability.

Dopamine A neurotransmitter that helps control physical movement (low amounts result in Parkinson's disease), improve mood (low amounts promote depression), sex drive, and retrieval of memory. It generally decreases with age, and lowered levels of dopamine have been linked to clinical depression.

Electroencephalogram (EEG) A test used to measure brain wave activity by placing electrodes on the outside of the head and measuring/recording the patterns of electrical activity that occur at certain locations.

Encoding The process of getting information into long-term memory. It involves a number of different mental tasks such as paying attention, reasoning something through, associating new information with other well-known and relevant information that already exists in long-term memory, analyzing information, and elaborating on details. Often these tasks are performed automatically without any conscious effort. They give deeper meaning to the information being considered and strengthen the chance that it will be remembered.

Endorphins A group of neurohormones released when the body experiences stress, or when we achieve a desired goal after efforts. They are "reward" chemicals that encourage motivation to continue doing some action or mental activity that is pleasurable. The structure of their molecules is similar to that of opiate drugs, and they are sometimes called endogenous opiates.

Engram A memory trace, or a structural change that takes place during learning and serves as the physiological substrate of memory.

Enzyme A protein that controls chemical reactions in living tissue.

Epinephrine A hormone secreted by the adrenal gland, which also acts as a neurotransmitter. The most powerful vasopressor or vasoconstrictor known, it raises blood pressure; controls bleeding; stimulates the heart muscle, accelerating heart rate; and by reducing the smooth muscles in the bronchii acts as a muscle relaxant during bronchial asthma attacks.

False memory syndrome   The recall of fictitious, usually traumatic, events, with the belief that the events are genuine.

Free radical   An oxygen molecule with an unpaired electron that is highly reactive, thus readily combining with other molecules, usually causing damage to them.

Gamma-aminobutyric acid (GABA)   A neurotransmitter believed to exert an inhibitory action on target cells. Blocking or inhibiting signal transmission helps to prevent nerve cells from firing too fast and overloading the system. GABA is necessary for sleep and relaxation; hence, people with low levels of GABA experience high levels of tension and anxiety. Many pharmaceutical sedatives and tranquilizers (Valium) attach to GABA receptors in the brain.

Ganglion (plural: ganglia)   A group of nerve-cell bodies existing outside the brain and spinal cord.

Glucocorticoid   A group of hormones produced by the adrenal cortex, some of which also may be produced synthetically, which aid in the transformation of carbohydrates into glucose, thereby raising the blood sugar level and general alertness. Glucocorticoids aid the release of amino acids from muscle, take fatty acids from fat stores, and increase the ability of muscles to tighten and avoid fatigue. Their release is triggered by a hormone of the pituitary.

Glucose   A simple sugar that derives from the breakdown of the foods we eat, and that is the principal source of energy for all the body's cells.

Gram (gm.)   A measurement of weight equal to approximately

1/28th of an ounce. Drugs and medications are measured in grams or portions of grams (see *milligrams* and *micrograms*).

Gray matter   Those portions of the central nervous system containing cell bodies. Although called "gray," its actual color is closer to tan (see also *white matter*).

Hippocampus   The curved, elongated ridge that forms the larger part of the olfactory cerebral cortex and is involved in memory storage and consolidation. The term comes from the Greek words for horse (*hippos*) and sea monster (*kampos*). Presumably the hippocampus derived its name because in cross-section, it resembles a sea horse.

Hormone   A chemical compound formed by certain glands and organs, which is absorbed into the blood and influences the functioning of other parts of the body.

Huntington's disease   A dementia that results in abnormal bodily movements, postures, and gaits.

Hypothalamus   A portion of the brain that regulates many aspects of metabolism, especially body temperature and hunger.

Ischemia   A sustained loss of blood pressure resulting in an insufficient amount of blood being delivered to a region of the body or to the brain (called "cerebral ischemia"). Ischemia affecting the heart or brain can cause a heart attack or a stroke.

Lecithin   A mixture of phospholipids that constitutes a major component of all living cells.

Lesion   Damage to cell tissue. When it occurs in the brain, it can alter behavior, learning, or the ability to remember.

Limbic system   The hippocampus, amygdala, and related structures that together help transform short-term memories into long-term ones. It is the system that transmits sensory perceptions, as well as pain, to the brain, and generates an emotional reaction to them.

Magnetic resonance imaging (MRI)   More sensitive than a CAT scan, this diagnostic and research technique uses strong magnetic fields to surround the head and bombard it with radio-frequency pulses. The brain emits signals that a computer then uses to develop pictures of the brain to measure brain activity.

Magnetic resonance spectroscopy imaging (MRSI)   A research technique that allows scientists to measure concentrations of substances in the brain.

Melatonin   A hormone of the pineal gland that regulates the sleep-wake cycle. It is secreted in response to darkness and has been linked to the regulation of circadian rhythms. It also produces lightening of the skin by causing the concentration of melanin in pigment-containing cells.

Membrane   See *cellular membrane*.

Metabolism   The body's normal process of turning food into energy.

Microgram (mcg.)   A measurement of weight that is equivalent to 1/1,000th of a milligram.

Milligram (mg.)   A measurement of weight equivalent to 1/1,000th of a gram (see *gram*).

Monamines   A group of amines (organic compounds derived from ammonia), some of which, such as serotonin, are important in transmission of messages in the neurons.

Monoamine oxidase (MAO)   An enzyme that is important because it performs the first step in the process of breaking down the amines formed in the body, beginning the chain of events that allows them to be metabolized and eliminated from the body. It serves to maintain the balance in the brain of chemical levels of important neurotransmitters. As we age, the levels of MAO increase, destroying more than its usual amount of amines and changing the balance between neurotransmitters, especially norepinephrine.

Nervous system   A collection of cells in the body that are specialized to transmit electrochemical information. It is commonly divided into the central nervous system, the peripheral or voluntary nervous system, and the autonomic or involuntary nervous system.

Neurobiology   The study of the structure, function, and chemistry of nerve cells (neurons) and of the aggregates of neurons that process information and initiate behaviors.

Neuron   The smallest anatomical unit of the nervous system, consisting of a cell body, dendrites, and an axon.

Neuroscientist   A scientist who studies the brain.

Neurotransmitter   A chemical substance that sends impulses (signals) across the synaptic gap from the axon of one neuron to the dendrites of another, thereby stimulating or inhibiting activity in the receiving neuron.

Norepinephrine   A hormone that also functions as a neurotransmitter, it can enhance memory performance and is released predominantly in response to hypotension (low blood pressure). Once released, it stimulates the capillaries to expand so that more blood can flow through the brain. It also causes the brain to be more alert, acting somewhat like an amphetamine to step up brain activity. It is vital to helping carry memories from short-term storage in the hippocampus to long-term storage in the neocortex. Commercially, it is known as Noradrenaline.

Organic memory disorders   Disorders having a physiological basis that may impair memory, such as a head injury, certain diseases, and toxic agents that have been taken into the body in some way (i.e., through the mouth, the skin, or by breathing).

Oxidation   A chemical reaction in which oxygen reacts with another substance, resulting in a chemical transformation. In many cases, this results in the formation of free radicals in the body.

Phosphatidylserine (PS), molecular structure   (See top of page 346 for molecular structure of PS.)

Phospholipids Molecules of fat in cell membranes.

Positron emission tomography (PET) An imaging technique that allows researchers to observe and measure brain activity by monitoring blood flow and concentration of substances, such as oxygen and glucose, in brain tissue.

Protein A molecule comprised of amino acids arranged in a specific order, which is determined genetically. Proteins include neurotransmitters, enzymes, and hundreds of other substances.

Recall Remembering information without clues being given.

Receptor A protein in a cell membrane that recognizes and binds to chemical messengers such as neurotransmitters.

Recognition Remembering information when clues are given.

Repression A controversial process that refers to the inability to recall extremely unpleasant memories or experiences.

Retrograde amnesia Difficulty remembering information or events that occurred prior to brain trauma.

Scopolamine A poisonous alkaloid found in various plants of the Solanaceae (nightshade) family, it is used to block neuronal transmission in the parasympathetic nervous system and as a central nervous system depressant. Accordingly, it has been used in combination with morphine as a sedative in surgery and obstetrics, and as a "truth serum." It is often used in laboratory animals to produce amnesia, in order to test "smart drugs" or antioxidants that might interfere with scopolamine's functioning.

Senile dementia An outdated term, previously used for dementia in old age and likely covering the symptoms now identified as Alzheimer's disease.

Serotonin An inhibitory neurotransmitter that is considered essential for relaxation, concentration, and sleep. It also plays a role in pain and mood regulation.

Short-term memory The retention of small amounts of information for about 30 seconds or less.

Suppression The forgetting of a memory by deliberately trying not to think about it.

Synapse or synaptic gap The multi-microscopic space that separates one neuron from others nearby and in which neurotransmitters are secreted and pass from one neuron to receptors in a neighboring neuron.

Synesthesia Where sensation in any one sensory modality (such as hearing) evokes a sensory experience in a second modality, like vision or touch.

Toxicity The quality of being affected by a poison or toxin. Toxic reactions in the body impair bodily functions, such as memory and learning, and damage cells.

Vasopressin A hormone secreted by the posterior lobe of the pituitary gland that can enhance memory, especially in individuals who have low blood pressure, since one of its functions is to raise blood pressure.

Vasopressor An agent that stimulates contraction of muscle tissues of the arteries and capillaries.

Vitamin Any of about 15 organic substances that are critical for life and health. Many vitamins cannot be manufactured by the body and so need to be supplied through dietary intake.

White matter Areas of the central nervous system comprised of nerve fibers, which appear white, as opposed to areas comprised of cell bodies, which appear gray or tan (see also *gray matter*).

INDEX

Note: Page numbers in *italics* indicate graphics.